PSYCHOTHERAPY WITH CHILDREN

A Desktop Manual ©

CHARLES A. SARNOFF, MD, DLFAPA, DLFAACP, DIPLOMATE ABP&N (P,ChP)

JON D SARNOFF, MD, MBA, FAAP DIPLOMATE AMERICAN BOARD OF PEDIATRICS..,

"When real life is wanting, one must create an illusion."

TCHEKOV

161 w61st St   New York, NY 10023

This volume is the final form of this book

BOOKS BY

CHARLES A. SARNOFF, M.D.

"LATENCY" BOOKS - Three Volumes

    VOLUME I   "LATENCY"

    VOLUME II   "PSYCHOTHERAPEUTIC STRATEGIES
                IN THE LATENCY YEARS"

    VOLUME III   "PSYCHOTHERAPEUTIC STRATEGIES
                IN LATE LATENCY THROUGH
                EARLY ADOLESCENCE"

SYMBOL BOOKS

"SYMBOLS IN STRUCTURE AND FUNCTION" - Three Volumes

    VOLUME I   "THEORIES OF SYMBOLISM"

    VOLUME II   "SYMBOLS IN PSYCHOTHERAPY"

    VOLUME III   "SYMBOLS IN CULTURE, ART, AND MYTH"

"THE FERAL SWAN" - A Novel

Maturation of the

symbolizing function of two men

shapes character and plot.

DESKTOP MANUAL OF CHILDHOOD PSYCHOTHERAPY ©
FOR: THERAPISTS, PEDIATRICIANS, AND PARENTS - FINAL FORM

Charles Sarnoff, MD
Jon Sarnoff, MD

To order additional copies of this book, contact:
Xlibris
1-888-795-4274
www.Xlibris.com
Orders@Xlibris.com
704158

TO: MAX AND MIA

LEE SARNOFF

TABLE OF CONTENTS

UNIT FOUR - THE MECHANISMS AND TECHNIQUE OF THERAPY

UNIT SIX - TERMINATION

UNIT SEVEN - LITERATURE............ 181

UNIT EIGHT - APPENDICES

CASE HISTORIES

INTRODUCTION

This is a treatise devoted to the dynamic psychotherapeutic treatment of children. In this therapy, talking and play are used to ameliorate disorders in adjustment.

JDS

WHAT IS PSYCHOTHERAPY?

CAS

Psychotherapy is a verbal technique that deals with pathological adjustment to stress, anxiety, and loss. Dynamic Psychotherapy for Children is distinguished from other therapies in that it seeks to identify and modulate the effects of unconscious influences on symptoms, moods, and behavior. Psychoanalytic insights make simple conversation insufficient for achieving this. To detect the effect of cognitive growth, and motivation in children, on symbol formation, planning, behavior, and unconscious fantasy, requires more than listening to and attending to verbal free association; something that may suffice for mature adults. Dynamic

Psychotherapy for children requires access to unconscious content expressed through cognitively age appropriate dreaming, play, and drawings, which is not readably available with children through verbal free association. The therapist's technique must be enhanced to include observation of the patient's play, art, and dreams in addition to verbalizations.

In dealing with a maturing child, therapeutic technique must constantly be tuned to fit maturational and developmental stages that are organized around fixations, and regressions. The therapist is alert to phase specific presentations of unconscious content into consciousness in the three phases of childhood, which are infancy, childhood and adolescence. These manifestations influence current phase behavior. If phase appropriate, they support phase normal behavior, and if modified by adaptation and maturity, bear the potential to become paradigms for the appropriate development of normal personalities. Or if unchanged, they intrude on later mental functioning, either through fixation or reactivation, imparting regressive immaturities to behavior.

Infancy and Early Childhood

FROM BIRTH TO 26 MONTHS

The experiences and recalls of a child this age are primarily physiological with word encoding and recall gradually increasing. Since there is no repression or symbols to contribute hidden meanings, dynamic psychotherapy has no role in treatment at this age. Treatment consists of the therapist advising the parents and caretakers and therapy sessions which offer opportunities for expression through play and corrective object relations.

The therapist can follow a child's thinking if he knows the potential limits to knowing that early cognition permits. The first sensations possibly detected by the child are haptic (internal). They are generated by physiological events. They are encoded in memory as physiological sensations. They are recognized as true when recalled for they represent the experience of true events. They are intrinsically as true as hunger, thirst, pain, longing, loneliness, and fear. By two and a half years of age, encoded memories increasingly consist of words, which are linked to haptic physiological sensations (see chart two in appendix). They represent ideas, which are linked to the strong sense of reality associated with linked physiological sensations.. When bourne to consciousness from memory, their expression, in the form of myths, are experienced as real. They do not give way to verbal influence. They have the form and characteristics of the slogans and concrete sound-bites, which in later life form the basis of group allegiances, and disparate truths that "clash by night" generating wars, and prejudice. Memory shapes the perception of the world.

The child's world-view, as transmitted to the therapist, is distorted by phase specific influences, which support irrational fears. When illusion, shaped by altered veritically tinged memory, crowds out reality, a distorted world awaits. The therapist is trained to be on the alert for affect linked words, which have entered consciousness, divorced from their latent meanings through distortion techniques. For instance the symbolizing function can mask unconscious meanings by creating new expressions in consciousness. Concrete thinking can also introduce altered expression through false substitutes, which have been equated to the original meanings solely through common predicates. Abstract thinking could enable the patient to identify and discredit such concrete linkages through the use of identities based on intrinsic characteristics. Ability to abstract does not become present till eight and a half years of age and truly effective until eleven years of age. This limits the use of confrontations and comparisons in interpretations by the therapist during early childhood.

In the early years of childhood (ending at eight and a half years) the identification of reality beyond the child's memory requires simple comments and techniques geared to the patient's ability to comprehend or process conflict. These include playing out in the transference, expansion of reported dreams, and in expression and discharge through play.

There are those, like numbers, which are neutral and respond only to being called forth, and there are words associated with affects and meanings that are constantly seeking mastery using distortion techniques, which enable their masked expression in conscious thought and mastery through behavior, play, and dreams. The task of the therapist is to trace out the original stresses that have been distorted and to address ways of dealing with them.

Therapeutic Relevance for Early childhood

Early on experience and encoding is physiological. Later recall of these entities are experienced as physiological and true. The addition of words creates encoded memory moieties consisting of words and affects. When remembered words refer to meanings apart from the body, the physiological sense of reality accompanies them. The recalls stand alone. They are seen to be external (visual-auditory telereceptor) perceptions. They are used to interpret new experiences and concepts, in terms of old beliefs with their strong sense of reality.

26 MONTHS TO FOUR YEARS

The ability to form symbols, which has variably been described as occurring as early as 18 or 26 months, should normally be present by 30 months. Dynamic Psychotherapy can be used in treating symbol based symptoms seen during this period. The symbols at this age are transparent. If asked, the child can tell the therapist, what the latent meaning of the symbol is. This introduces explorations of the stresses the child is facing, providing the possibility of mastery through venting for the child and information for advising the parents and care takers about changes in management.

The content of psychopathology during the 30 months (See Sarnoff) to 48 months (See Piaget) period relates to the establishment of a boundary between the self and the world, projection across this boundary which produces night fears of threatening figures in the dark, paranoia and the lock in of life influencing conflicts and fantasies, all felt to be real. Expressed through manifest symbols, the latter consist of myths, fantasies and the imposed endowed truths of religion. These elements are encoded using concrete verbal memory during the period of acquisition of concrete ideas through speech. They are supported by the sense of reality to be unchallengeable truth. Such engendered truths persist uneroded in unconscious memory. Related conflicts, drives, and conscious manifestations either are held in repression or persist as fixations. The conscious sound bites that represent concrete verbal memory encoding are unchallengeable, No argument can be introduced in confronting these beliefs. They are two dimensional- The conflicts they hide are beyond the reach of logic.

During the transition period involving early individuation, emphasis shifts from haptic experience to the telereceptor experience of outside non self entities. A boundary is created across which primitive projection can occur. Perceptions are displaced and assigned to the differentiated external part of the experience. Discomforts, anger, erotic sensations, can be assigned to a non-self 'other" such as a dark shadowy figure in the night.

FROM FOUR YEARS TO SIX YEARS

The advent of repression (See Piaget), which becomes
stronger over these two years, makes the uncovering
of symbolic meanings so difficult that emphasis in
therapy must be added to the use of mastery through
play, drawings and dream expansion. Symbols and
words at this age, whose meanings have no abstract
facets to use when exploring for an expansion of
meaning contributes an uncontestable element to the
child's thinking. Being immune to challenge, they
become the paradigmatic model for paranoia. Crowds
of symbols mark the place where the secrets of drive
impelled fantasies lie hidden in memory. Search
for latent content is impaired by the capacity of
symbols to mask meaning, leaving only glancing hints
from dreams. Our search for unconscious motivation
through related word meanings is made difficult
by the absence of abstract facets and unchanging
content in the meanings and definitions of words used
as symbols at this age. The existence of projected
persecutors in paranoid episodes can be identified
by the unchanging symbolic content that is repeated
in one (paranoid) episode after another. Though
verbal interpretations of unconscious content,
motivations, and repressed traumas are an important
part of the psychotherapeutic technique for this
age, resolution of symptoms is also achieved by a
transition to latency defenses (see below), change
in fantasy content, the

THE LATENCY AGE CHILD - 6 to 12 years of age.

The latency age child is held suspended between restless desires and ambitions, and the limitations of his body. Drives are present, but not as strong as the flooding power that will be acquired with adolescence. With no sexual outlet for sexual drives and being too small to fight adults or bullies, he is a "biologically soldier dwarf" One child answered the question "What's wrong with being a child" with this description of the experience, "How would you like to be eight years old and not have a dime to your name?"

When real life is wanting as a means of adjusting to needs and reality, the latency age child, hobbled by the realities of his immaturity, creates fantasy-illusions as an adjustment. There is a mobilization of neutral energies in the service of calmness, cooperativeness and educability, This activity is supported by the mobilization of fantasy about future planning, athletics, and identity. Under the impact of stresses such as being bullied, exposed to nudity, humiliation, and punishment, regression to anal level defense dominated fantasy takes place. Fantasies of world destruction, stealing, and revenge are developed. Most latency age children are brought to treatment because they have been acting on these fantasies. The most adaptive response is the regression to aggressive fantasy, which is defended against by reaction formations in the form of calm, quiet cooperativeness.

At about eight and a half years of age interpretations using abstractions become possible. This resource becomes stronger until eleven years of age when proverb interpretation becomes a normal skill. A change in persecutory figures in the fear and persecutory fantasies of children transition from amorphous figures to humanoid ones at eight and a half years of age. This is not the product of therapy. It is a result of maturation. In spite of the fact that latency fantasy supports states of latency and should be encouraged to protect the child so he can grow and be prepared for involvement with the world during adolescence, the defense oriented antisocial fantasies of latency should be analyzed in order to avert current social problems and future aberrant adjustment difficulties. Regression to or fixation at latency age adjustment influences the form that psychopathology takes during adolescence and adulthood. Should illusion inform self-image and action, and persist as a powerful affect laden memory, expression through pathological symptom formation and aberrant behavior can be expected.

Maturation and development contribute to growth, behavioral improvement and adjustment during childhood. Spontaneous improvement may be expected with the advent of adolescence. Appraisal of the curative role of psychotherapeutic treatment in childhood should take into account the expected effect of maturation. Pedagogic therapeutic techniques may be needed to fulfill the development of potentials opened for the child by maturation.

ADOLESCENCE-

Adolescence is most often associated with the increase in the flow and force of sexual hormones that activate sexual characteristics during puberty. The beginning of adolescence is characterized during a psychotherapy by a gradual shift of the session venue from the playroom with its play and toys to one's consultation room with emphasis on verbal exchange, reporting, and free association. This occurs with both boys and girls. For girls, puberty brings an increase in verbalization. It is said that one can tell, when menarche begins, by increase in verbalization. A direction of attention to the finding of a sexual partner for girls arises as a concern for the male therapist. Acting out of a transference involving the therapist, with a classmate or a sexual predator, should be explored and interpreted to the patient. At first love fantasies in adolescence have the characteristics of self-centered Hollywood partnering. At about fifteen, the adolescent love fantasy involves knowing the loved one and exploring and participating in teamwork.

The symbols of children of latency age or younger are called ludic symbols. Ludic means play. Ludic symbols give fantasies the power to express and work through conflicts and stresses through expression in play dreams and fantasy. Permitting a child patient to play out fantasies during sessions is a therapeutic activity. The onset of adolescence is forced by ludic demise, when the symbols lose the capacity to serve in place of a real person. In adolescence object seeking cathexes shift from the no longer effective humanoid ludic symbols of late latency fantasies to real people.

During adolescent contacts with the un-giving stress producing demands of reality and the world, the child acquires the ability to deal with unexpected pressures. One of the most important tasks of adolescence is the acquisition of the ability to deal with stress. If protective parents or substance abuse interfere with these skills, an incompetent adult will be the result. Mastery of stress without chemical avoidance strategies is an important part of the therapy of the adolescent. Adolescence ends at the brink of marriage and career. It is never too early to emphasize due diligence in the selection of a college, a career, or a spouse. An example is the admonition know whom are marrying before you marry her.

JDS WHAT IS PSYCHOTHERAPY?

CAS Psychotherapy is a treatment technique that deals with pathological adjustment to stress, anxiety, and loss. It is as old as dream interpretation, and comfort offered to a friend. Theseus offered therapy to Oedipus in "Oedipus at Colonus"

There are many forms of "talking based help" used in treating troubled children. Dynamic Psychotherapy for Children, as presented here, is distinguished from other verbal therapies in that it seeks to identify and modulate the effects of unconscious influences on symptoms, moods, and behavior. Freudian insights into the effect of cognitive growth, unconscious fantasy, and motivation, on behavior and symbol formation, make simple conversation insufficient. In Dynamic Psychotherapy for children, the therapist's technique is enhanced to include ways of accessing unconscious content that is not readably available through verbal free association or questioning. It places emphasis on patient observation, play, and art as well as verbalization and dream interpretation during therapist-patient communication. For a child, with ongoing maturation the therapy is adjusted to fit a multitude of maturational and developmental stages. The therapist's approach must constantly be tuned to fixations, regressions, and ongoing shifts to new phases, reflecting age appropriate maturity. The therapist must be alert to regressions to earlier levels of function. Variations in technique are introduced to fit the developmental characteristic of the age phase of the child. These phases are infancy (preverbal), early childhood (verbal) (symbolic after 2 1/2yrs.), latency age (concrete symbolic - Abstract after 8 1/2) and adolescence. When working with adults, there seems to be a fixed maturity level to work with. The phases of the adult are few. The phases of the child are as many as his days.

Pathological adjustment occurs when ideas and fantasies in memory arise to consciousness in the form of ideas and opinions that alter the perception of reality. The role of the therapist is to clear the way to reality perception by identifying such distortions of imagery.

There are two sources of memory content. These are the encoding of perception and experience from the earliest moments of life, and the acquisition of endowed knowledge (St. Thomas Aquinas) through parental and pastoral teaching and spiritual experience. The two realities described are responsible for two types of psychotherapy. The first, dynamic psychotherapy, deals with the influence on adjustment and behavior of memory encoded from perceived reality. The second, Analytic Psychology and pastoral guidance interpret also the influence of religious teaching, and a flow into memory from a universal knowledge base that exists independently of the brains of living men. Intrusions from this knowledge base can take the form of a dream. Pastoral guidance perceives dreams as pathways for the will of deity, seen as a guide to proper life choices. The dynamic psychotherapist must be alert to influential endowed memory elements that shape life choices and adjustment. Dynamic Child Therapy is best done without challenges to these beliefs, for these beliefs are part of the mortar that shapes and holds together the family.

UNIT ONE-

THE SETTING

CHANCE AND THE PREPARED PLAYROOM HELP THERAPY
PROGRESS

PLAYROOM, AND OFFICE FLOOR-PLANS

There are two types of floor-plans for an office to be used for child therapy. There is the adaptation of a single room office designed for the psychotherapy of adults, and there is the multi-room office designed specifically with the needs of children, in dynamic child therapy, in mind.

Adapting a single room office
to the needs of
Dynamic Child Therapy

Minimally that which is required for child therapy, is a waiting area, a consultation room, and a bathroom. Typically the waiting area contains a few chairs, a table to hold reading material and access to the bathroom. The waiting and the consultation room should be separated by some sound proofing. One such consultation room, that I remember well was furnished with an office desk that was used for drawing and building, a drawer for holding toys, clay, and drawing materials, adult sized chairs that fit the desk, an analytic couch, a floor rug, and a three foot high multicolor wooden Danish soldier figure placed in the office to provide atmosphere.

If such an office room is on a low floor, window access to distracting sounds and sights should be minimized through use of draperies.

Such an office should work for a highly talented and well trained therapist. Financial considerations, sometimes makes it essential to use such a setting. For those whose motivation is to fill a few afternoon hours or to work toward a new credential, it is held forth to be enough.

Multi-room offices
designed specifically for
Dynamic Child Therapy.

Childhood psychopathology has many facets. Treatment needs to adapt. More than one room is required if one is to explore the many ways, through many phases that the developing child uses to express and master encoded affect laden experiences held in memory.

When recommending my book "Latency" to students, an instructor advised them not to expect the striking clinical experiences reported in the book. But they happened. I attribute their presence to variable settings that enhance the ability to perceive and create swiftly changing forms of symbolic expression; words, play, pictures, dreams. As swift as thought, these forms can interchange in a single session. There is no time to refurnish a room. For example: the late-latency-adolescent child, who shifts between play and talk therapy, can move easily between a playroom and a consultation room, leaving or seeking distractions as he wills. A single room can be reorganized in advance to adapt the therapeutic approach to fixed age related changes in the symbols produced by the developing ego.

Multi-room offices for use in Dynamic Child Therapy require a waiting room, a patient's bathroom, a consultation room with bathroom and near playroom access. Playrooms should offer easy access to the consultation room, and the bathroom. An independent small business office for record keeping, billing, and filing is pleasant to have.

The waiting area contains a couch, a few chairs, a table to hold reading material. A separate room off the vestibule is ideal to assure patients privacy. This doesn't always work. Jimmy was a curious 14 year old lad, who always looked into the waiting room before leaving the office. Access to the bathroom, associated with the waiting room, should be easy. A place for hanging winter clothes should be available in the vestibule.

The waiting and the consultation rooms should be separated by some sound proofing. The consultation room should not be crowded with furniture. Few and neutral pictures should adorn the walls. An office desk should be set into the room. Its back should be far enough away from the wall behind it for the therapist's chair to be pulled away from the desk, permitting easy exit out of the desk chair. A clear exit path between the therapist and the patient from the chair to a door is a safety feature. Its presence is an expression of the conclusion that foresight is better than hind sight. Psychotherapy is not considered to be dangerous. Patients tend to hurt non-medical therapists, not physicians.

Therapists should be prepared and ever alert. Why? Here are four cases.

Hermine von Hug-Helmuth was the first women to earn a PhD from the University of Vienna. She became interested in Freud's work, became a psychoanalyst and became the first person to use play therapy in the practice of Child Analysis. Essentially she founded the field. She had a nephew, Rolf, whom she had helped to raise. She developed theory based on her work with him as a patient. In 1924, when Rolf was 18 years old, he murdered her; by strangulation.

A Swiss biologist, who had earned his PhD with a study of the molusks of Lake Leman, decided to follow his sister and become a psychoanalyst. He became a teaching analyst and even met with Freud to discuss his work on the origin of symbols in childhood. One of his first patients caused him to shift from analysis to the developmental study of childhood cognition. In the first sessions of analysis with that patient on the couch, he thought to himself that "This man has mean friends." Soon the patient came to the session bearing a dangerous weapon. The analysis was terminated. It is a good idea to have enough background in psychiatric differential diagnosis to identify paranoia, schizophrenia, and a tendency to act out fantasies generated by dynamic treatment.

I have been an infectious disease physician, a psychiatrist, and a research flight surgeon. I do

not seek danger. It sits on my shoulder. An office
with an available safety exit is reassuring for
me. Jennie was eighteen, a lovely blue eyed blond
schizophrenic. After a consultation, I met with her
parents. I explained my findings and the necessary
therapeutic plan. Hospitalization was presented as
a resource. The father rose shaking with rage. He
moved threateningly toward me, muttering that his
mother had been hospitalized for schizophrenia,
implying that psychiatrists were responsible. His
wife interposed herself; saving me injury.

In a 400 bed psychiatric hospital, a seminar was
being held. I was sent to find and escort a patient
to the seminar for presentation. I had examined the
patient once before. He responded to my greeting
with the declaration that," You remind me of my
butcher. I'm going to kill you." I retreated to the
seminar. The head of department advised me to avoid
the patient and reassigned him to a new doctor...

A little advance planning helps.

If the consultation office room is on a low floor,
window access to distracting sounds and sights
should be minimized through use of draperies or
glassing-in of the street facing wall. Investigate
before you sign the lease to be sure that the
apartment above you is not occupied by a piano
teacher. A small refrigerator can be useful. A
couch, chair, diplomas and a bookcase are commonly
present.

There are two types of playrooms.

One is small (10 feet by 10 feet). It has linoleum flooring. There is a table with two child size chairs. One of the chairs has a broad seat and shorter legs than its partner chair. This chair facilitates comfortable seating for a therapist's relatively large posterior and places the therapists head near to level with that of the child. Shelves for large pieces of paper, clay, pencils, and markers should be on one wall, Avoid paint which could splatter and make a big mess. Note that the independent physical status of the playroom makes it possible to delay the cleaning up of messes. Water play may be indicated. Some therapists keep a bottle of water in the playroom. A sink connected to plumbing is contraindicated. A child may insinuate himself between the sink and the therapist, block the faucet with his finger, and send a spray that soaks him. To solve this problem, install a camper's pump sink or have an extra shirt ready. Individual cubbies which close out the curious are useful for the safekeeping of projects between sessions. One wall should be of cork to hold drawings. Another should be plastic coated for writing on the wall that can be cleaned.

The second playroom has a rug, is larger than the first room, and is more comfortable to use while sitting on the floor with a child who is playing out a fantasy. Since it can be large, one must keep in mind that the child may be using the extra space to position herself in a way that interferes with the therapist's view of what she is doing. This maneuver can be countered by creating a play story with ludic symbols (toys, cut-outs) that will attract the patient's attention. The scenario should sufficiently vague that when, the child asks what one is doing, one can say "What do you think", bringing the theme of the session back to what is on the child's mind. Like the smaller room, therapy is facilitated by a child height workbench table that can be used for drawing and building with small chairs one of which has a broad seat. A private cubby for each child in treatment can preserve works in progress and themes worth revisiting. A drawer for holding toys, clay, and drawing materials should be near at hand. There are therapists who recommend that there be a drawer for cookies for the patient. I am not one of them. Oral needs should be listened for, focused, and analyzed; not fed. Sharp tools like scissors require special attention. Young children do not understand the limits that apply to knives and sharp pointed scissors. If scissors are needed for construction, blunt nose scissors are safer. Eternal vigilance must be maintained. There is no place for sharps in a therapy session. There is no place for lighters either. If a child of any age brings such items to the session, early blocking of acting in is required. Once a child begins to act physically, it is too late. I prefer to say, "Whatever you want to do, put it into words. Action could hurt. I'm here to protect you from action." A young teenager, known for 'hocking a lugie' was proud of his role in school theatricals. He proudly spoke of his classmate's bewildered reaction to "being rained on" with thick mucous raindrops. This history alerted me to the potential implied by his opening the window, looking down at the cars in the parking lot, gathering many sheets of paper near the window, and displaying a cigarette lighter that he had found that day in school. I identified his possible future action and said, "Don't even think of it." His impetus to action deflated, he turned to words.

The choice between type of play room usually is determined by availability. What is important is that the child friendly setting encourages abreaction through fantasy play or art, and that the child be treated with respect.

... PLAY THERAPY and the TELEPHONE

Stopping a therapy to answer the telephone distracts the therapist's attention, admits to a therapist priority that ignores a patient's needs, interferes with fantasy insight and continuity, and wastes therapy time. Sometime it is welcomed by the patient as a help in resisting treatment. A telephone held in a desk drawer with absent tone and a flickering call signal light out of the patient's sight makes it possible to avoid interrupting a treatment, and yet be ready to pick up or answer calls between sessions.

What if something important has happened to the child that a parent wants the therapist to know? 0A break between sessions affords one the opportunity to pick up messages from an answering machine placed between the consultation room and the playroom. This arrangement can be valuable for dreams. Children dream and report the dreams to their parents. Often the force of the dream has been dissipated by its telling to the point that it is not recalled in the therapy session. Parents can counter this by leaving a dream report on the answering machine. The therapist informed by the light signal can pick up the dream and be alerted to listen for an important topic during the next session, before it begins. "Did something happen to you last night while you were sleeping?." If not used too often this intervention can effectively bring the dream into the therapy session.

Psychotherapy with children requires an environment that gives priority to the child, his feelings and his thoughts. The child is best served in a room set aside for play. The room should be at most ten feet by ten feet. If there is a window, it should open onto a quiet place, such as an enclosed garden. A view of the doors of a firehouse would be too distracting. An enclosing curtain should be available for use in excluding distractions. A mess left after play can happen. A corner of one's consulting room can thus not serve, for the mess, a useful self expression for the child, would make the room of little use in dealing with an adult in the next session. Taking the therapy into the open air imperils the therapy. A passing frightened squirrel, followed by a distracted child patient, pursued by a distressed child therapist, creates a context that discourages insight.

TOILETS

The number and location of toilets in facilities needed for use in the private practice of the dynamic psychotherapy of children are manifold. They are the products of the opinions of the deciding practitioner and his recall of the needs and inclinations of parents and patients.

I have found that two toilets are best to have. One should be connected to the office. One should be connected to the waiting room area. This preference is derived from sixty plus years of practice experience and an equivalent number of years listening to the experiences of colleagues. There is no general agreement on this issue. I therefore have decided to include here case histories illustrating related needs and approaches, to be used as guides..

Dr. Bill was in his early thirties. He was a psychoanalytic candidate. A supervisee in training with him was shown his office. One closet, when opened, was filled to the brim with toilet paper. Dr. Bill announced, "You can't have enough". That was the year that Dr. Bill was dropped from his training institute.

Recommendation – Obsessional overemphasis on bathroom cleanliness should be considered to be beyond the call of duty. However out of a sense of courtesy to those who will require a waiting room toilet, especially for practices with over ten patients a day, an adequate supply of toilet paper should be available. Resorting to a toilet paper caddy, capable of holding over two rolls, hung on the toilet, has served me well. Toilet paper theft has not been an issue. The same goes for soap and towels.

Mrs. S.B. was a forty year old mother of an overactive non-achieving nine year old boy in treatment with me. She and her husband were waiting for a meeting with me to discuss her son's therapy. When I came into the waiting area of the ground floor office beneath my home, I found her husband; hovering over her and expressing concern. Her eyes were filled with rage. She shouted at him, "I have to go! I refuse to go up these stairs to use a bathroom in the house." He quaked. I interrupted her with a gesture toward a nearby door. "That's the waiting room bathroom.", said I.

Recommendation – The waiting room bathroom should be clearly marked.

Dr. J.C. was a young adult-psychoanalytic teacher assigned to teach residents, of which I was one. He had recently bought a brownstone house. He had renovated the ground floor. He proudly showed us the two bathrooms he had added. One was attached to his consultation room. Said he, "It's a relief not to have to share the patient's bathroom." He spoke of avoiding embarrassment.

Comment - In sixty plus years, I have had to respond to an emunctory crisis twice. Each time, I explained the ensuing interruption, and used the waiting room bathroom. I could not detect any impact on the ongoing treatment. For evacuative embarrassment, some additional analysis of the analyst might be indicated.

Ms. J. L. was a high school student who came directly from school. When I entered the waiting room to greet her. She announced that the waiting room bathroom could not be used. The ceiling had fallen down. I looked. She was right. I directed her to the second bathroom that was off my consulting room.

Recommendation - In an old building, check the status of the bathroom ceiling, before you sign the lease.

Ms. J. M. was a high school student, who came to sessions early and did home-work while waiting for me. One day, I came out to great her, only to find her books, but no patient in the waiting room. Precisely at the moment her session was scheduled to start, the bathroom door opened. There she was. She demanded to start the session immediately. A shy smile preceded her demand. She wanted to know if I needed the bathroom. She began the session by telling of her fantasy that she had put me in an embarrassing situation.

Comment – The usefulness of a separate consulting room bathroom is clearly illustrated here.

DR. R.L. had recently graduated from adult and child Psychoanalytic training. He moved into a prewar apartment above a restaurant in Manhattan. One room was used as a consulting room. The small vestibule near the entrance door was used as a waiting room. There was no bathroom in the apartment for patient use. When asked about this by his colleagues, he replied, "They can use the bathroom in the restaurant downstairs."

Comment –Minimally, professional considerations require that we consider the comfort of our patients. There are also safety features, which are discussed in the office floor-plan section.

Privacy and toileting are linked concepts. A door that can be locked is a natural feature of a bathroom opening to a public space. In my experience only a lock with a pushbutton facing in and a keyhole equipped knob facing out is adequate for the needs of the child therapist's office. The pushbutton can lock in responds to the light touch of a small child. The keyhole outer knob can be used by an adult swiftly to open a door that has been locked and stayed locked either as a child's malign power gesture, or as an expression of ignorance.

The preferred bathroom facilities, would be two bathrooms; one of which has access from the consultation room; the other, which should be clearly marked, should be in immediate contact with the waiting room. Soap and tissues should be available in good supply. Doors should have push button inside locks, which can be easily opened by an adult.

UNIT TWO –

THE PARTICIPANTS

NO CHILD IS AN ISLAND.

NO ONE EVER CAN STAND SO TALL

AS ONE WHO STOOPS TO HELP A CHILD

THE ROLE OF PARENTS IN THERAPY

The parent's role is to support therapy. For instance, parents learn to say "Why not talk to the doctor about this? He may have some good ideas." Parents serve therapy in ways that the child is not ready to undertake. Children have no advance readiness for using a professional in the handling of adjustment problems. One cannot expect a child to report on dreams, personal problems, parental discipline, or stresses. All that one can expect to work with at the beginning of therapy, with a child, is his ability to play, symbolize, remember, and create fantasy; complicated by defenses, such as repression and symbol formation, that obscure memory content. Presentation of the child's experiences, the exposition of his history. and reports on his current experiences require the input of parents, teachers and caretakers. Sessions and telephone contacts with parents are necessary if the therapist is to get the whole picture. Access to an answering machine near the playroom can serve well to enable the reporting of dreams, events, and the future plans and events. Cordless I-phones without ringers serve this purpose well.

Dreams often contain messages for the patient's customary dream interpreter; the parent. After being told to the parent, the dream is lost and is forgotten; its energy for communication having been lessened. Thus telling dreams to parents diverts them from presentation in therapy sessions. The parent often must serve as a dream bearer via telephone.

The child learns to understand the role of the therapist and begins direct dream reporting to him in response to questions, phrased in terms of a child's experience. "Did something happen to you when you were sleeping last night?" is better than "What did you dream last night?"

The child-parent couple-hood carries in it early man's need for a companion, at home and while traveling, who will serve as a dream interpreter. Oedipus told his wife his dreams. Pharaoh told his dreams to Joseph. Gilgamesh brought his dreams to his mother, when at home. While traveling he turned to his friend Enkidu, whose loss was devastating. In ancient Egypt and Greece there were professional dream interpreters. They worked fairs. They pondered the meaning of dreams. Artemadorus of Daldus, who traveled to the fairs of the ancient world interpreting dreams, instructed his son in the profession of dream interpreting. In his book about dream meanings "The Interpretation of Dreams" he advised against interpreting irrational content in dreams (20%); for "No one will ever make a living interpreting that.").

It is not wise to reveal that the privacy, enjoyed by the child and the parent-interpreter, has been betrayed by the parent through a reporting phone call to the therapist. The dream of a child could lose power to carry secrets. It would be better to ask about the topic introduced in a phone call about a dream, or to be guided by the dream content to focus on related content that appears during therapeutic play. For instance a three person dream containing a threat to the child could suggest that the therapist introduce dolls or clay figures to be used in play. An oedipal fear fantasy involving parental equivalents could evolve. This approach can be used by therapists working with children who have not yet reached the capacity to get the main idea from a narrative or a dream. Endlessly detailed goalless reports of dreams, as long as twenty minutes, occur,. The therapist can select play-things offered as a way of focusing on a content aspect of an endless dream.

There are situations in which parents, who are threatened by the child's growing skills, will put down a child; undermining the child's self image and his courage to interface with reality. Such children regress to fantasy. If possible the parent who undermines a child's spirit should be influenced to stop. There are parents whose feelings are so deep that they cannot do this. For instance a professional man diverted attention from a question about his feelings for his son (an eight year old thief, who had recently stolen gold from a neighbor.) by telling me this "joke".

"Once there was a man, who wanted to know what it felt like to have a baby.

He blocked his outlet with a cork.

After many months he was so hot and uncomfortable that he sat in the bleachers of a baseball game naked.

A curious monkey noted the plug as he ambled by. He pulled it out.

The down-flow engulfed him.

The man observed the coated being..

The man said, "I don't care if you are a piece of s—t, you're mine and I love you."

The family situation may reflect this kind of thinking; the therapy and therapist being often undercut. If, as in the case of this father, direct intervention with the father was ineffectual, introduction of skill enhancing, self image improving constructions, such as models, were useful. The father could not change. He had need to diminish all whom he met. For instance, when the child was seeking a profession upon graduating from college, the parents sought my guidance. "What have you considered as appropriate for him?" asked I. Said the father, "My wife thinks he should be a lawyer. I don't think so. That takes a real man. I think he should do something like what you do."

Symptoms in a child from such a family hover about low self image, uncertainty about convictions, and a sense of inadequacy. Interpretation or verbal reassurance is not a useful means for confronting these feelings. Insight helps little. Action and corrective object relations in the therapy supports the enhancement of self image.. If the child gets a 90% grade on a test, "Where are the other 20 points?", is out of place. Letting the child win board games is appropriate here. The making of model planes, boats, and electronic instruments can be the basis for the development of a self image supportive of living a life independent of the father's needs.

Identifying Progress

From the start, to work as a team, parent therapist contacts should be influenced by the parental view of what therapy is and can do. Parents expect perfection. Discuss what the problems are, and what signs and symptoms need to be resolved,. Once these are identified, one can ask about improvement as the therapy progresses, as a clinical focus of attention. Most parents do not have experience with therapy and do not know how to identify progress toward termination. For example, a parent of a disruptive child asked, when the child became cooperative, why therapy could not be ended abruptly, "You have good results, why look for perfect results?", asked the father. He did not realize that the signs and symptoms of childhood psychopathology change, like the mistletoe, with time and the season. These signs and symptoms can even disappear when the child transitions into a new age period. For instance neurotic obsessive-compulsive behavior fades out as adolescence fades in. Clearing up of age related immediate current symptomatic events and problems can occur without the resolution of underlying character patterns, such as overaggressive fantasies, longings, and persisting immature defenses. Resolving underlying character patterns can avert return of symptoms and future difficulties, such as the generation of age appropriate pathology as a reaction to the burgeoning hormonal activity of puberty. Persistence of certainty laced projection underlies the transition from night fears and infantile zoophobias at five years of age to adult agoraphobic fears. That such future difficulties can be avoided through psychotherapy should be identified to parents early in the treatment. That clearing the symptom does not clear the underlying psychopathology should also be included. The presence of infantile psychopathology is an early warning sign that there will be psychological difficulties in later life. Treatment offers, to the child, whose intense fantasy life interferes with attention at school, resorbtion of the conflictual underpinnings that support distracting mental content.

FEES

Fees to be paid for therapy are an unavoidable topic for discussion during the first meeting with parents. Young families often have many children and many bills to pay. Psychotherapeutic sessions are expensive. As soon as is possible, it should be determined if the family can afford therapy. Set the fee before parents get involved so that alternative plans can be discussed. Otherwise the

parents may feel forced to reject any therapy,
to the child's detriment. For sessions reserved
for work with children and adolescence, flexible
pricing can offer to the therapist an opportunity
to work with a broader variety of cases in the
future. Enhanced experience offers enhanced skills,
with better results with patients in the future. In
my own case, I spent gainful many years offering
consultation and morning psychotherapy sessions
at an eight hundred child normal child caring
institution (orphanage).

CONSULTATION OR THERAPY

Consultation in child psychiatry consists of three
parts, initial meeting with parents, a diagnostic
examination with the child, and a final reporting
session, with a report to be prepared. Therapy if
needed, is initiated after the third meeting. The
situation contains pitfalls. To avoid three unpaid
sessions and preparation of a report, the parent
should be told at first contact that it is customary
to pay for two of the sessions during the first
meeting and for the last session at that meeting.
Parents of children, subject to school referred
consultations, tend to avoid payment. Before one
takes on a consultation, one should be sure that
you can follow up with therapy if needed. If not,
the situation should be explained to the parents.
In this way multiple consultations can be avoided.
The pitfall in this situation is illustrated in
this episode. I went into the waiting room to get
the child to bring him to the consultation room.
He was slow to follow me. He began to cry.. Said he

"This is my seventh time. At first the doctor likes me, but after he gets to know me, he doesn't want to see me." This is an avoidable situation. If one is to recommend treatment, one should be ready to give treatment.

THE TEACHER'S ROLE

Teachers and caretakers are importantly involved with the lives of child patients. Much time away from parents is spent with them. Information about behavior and development unnoticed by parents can be missed if teachers are not involved in the work of therapy. Contact with the teacher should be initiated as soon as possible. A mutual exchange of contact information is an important goal. Because the schedules of teachers and child psychiatrists make contact during the day difficult, home phone numbers are essential to setting up a functioning ongoing contact. The time of the beginning of the patient's sessions should be given to the teacher so that she can leave up to the minute reports of importance relating to dreams, newly introduced academic topics, regressions, embarrassments etc., on the office voicemail telephone system. Most teachers cooperate. Some feel that the child therapist is an intruder into her world.

Not infrequently a teacher lets the therapist know that she cannot understand why such a lovely and well behaved child is seeing a therapist and dismisses you haughtily. Wait! For the brain damaged child,

disruptive behavior in the classroom begins a few
days or immediately after transfer or initiation of
contact with a new classroom. For the emotionally
disturbed child, wait! It may take a few weeks before
the teacher calls to ask for help in handling your
mutual patient. It takes that long for the child to
get the lay of the land, to find out other's weak
spots, and discover who is ripe for some neurotic
interaction in the classroom.

WHAT THE THERAPIST NEEDS TO KNOW

A backdrop of changing contexts, must be considered
by a child therapist when identifying pathology
and when developing psychotherapeutic strategies.
Therapists who work with children must adjust their
therapeutic approaches, thinking, and interventions
to the encoding, recording, and remembering
cognitive skills that are appropriate for the
patient's age. One cannot expect from a child
teamwork or appreciation of the benefits offered
by a professional in resolving emotional problems,
until a child is fifteen years of age.

Parents bring the child for psychotherapy. Children
are willing to play. They can hardly be expected
to understand the role of unconscious motivation
in their behavior or to cooperate directly with
the therapist. For example, Fred was five years
old. His mother's chief complaint was that his
behavior was motivated by the question, "Who is
the boss of me?". At the start of a session he told
me, "A funny thing happened when I came through
the door downstairs. I got all better." Through

application of his knowledge of child development, especially in regard to the influence of encoded memories on childhood comprehension, the therapist brings therapy to the child. Knowledge of the pitfalls introduced to development described above enables the pediatrician to support the therapist, when developmental changes introduce unexpected activity.

THE GROWING CHILD

THERAPEUTIC TECHNIQUE UNDERGOES CONTINUOUS MODIFICATION THAT ADAPTS IT TO ONGOING MATURATIONAL AND DEVELOPMENTAL CHANGES IN THE GROWING CHILD.

GROWTH IS ACCOMPANIED BY CHANGE IN TECHNIQUES OF MEMORY ENCODING, AGE AND SIZE, AVAILABLE LOVE OBJECTS, SYMBOLIZING SKILLS, COGNITION, AND CAPACITY FOR ABSTRACT THINKING.

MEMORY ONTOGENESIS

THE STAGE OF MEMORY ENCODING SHAPES COGNITION

Of the many factors that contribute to neurotic symptomatology, reminiscence is foremost. As Freud (1897) described it "Neurotics suffer mainly from reminiscences." (p. 244). Other determining factors are ambient expectations, growing and changing cognition, and, shaping influences of readiness for encoding that mature with age.

Each reminiscence consists of three phases. These are:

1. Source (origin),

2. Encodings (stored memories)

3. Representations (recalled memories).

A metaphor for this breakdown into elements can be found in describing the phases through which gold transitions on its way from lava to jewelry. These are:

1. Source (an element extruded from a volcano)

2. Ore (storage in the earth)

3. Jewelry (shaped into a ring, a rememberable form).

Sources remain constant over the years. The means of encoding in memory alters in keeping with maturational changes that accompany the passing years. Once encoded, a memory can move back and forth between a stored form and a recalled form. Representations are influenced by customs and styles.

STAGES OF MEMORY ENCODING FROM BIRTH THROUGH EIGHT YEARS OF AGE

Each stage of maturational development has specific memory encoding characteristics. Pathology in later years can be identified through finding memory encoding features that are appropriate for earlier years.

Infantile fixations and regressions in the patient, either reported by parents or that occur as responses to stress in the therapy, should alert the child therapist to the presence of underlying content of psychotherapeutic value. Evidence of fixation indicates immaturity and sustained impaired parenting. For instance encopresis (recalled in action) at seven should suggest that parental expectations and discipline should be explored. Parental expectations should grow apace; keeping ahead of the child's growth. The presence of regressive characteristics may indicate the existence of a current stress. For instance, the sobbing of an eight year old before a test is a regressive response that can be related to infancy by explorations of the child's coping mechanisms. Waking parents at night because of anxiety about tomorrow's dress could indicate little capacity to delay through the use of deflecting fantasy using symbol formation. This would require therapeutic techniques that enhance symbol formation. (see treating "asymbolia" below.)

LIST OF STAGES IN THE DEVELOPMENT OF ENCODING IN MEMORY

Stage 1   Physiological memory

Stage 1a. Preverbal - dominates first two years - encoding through muscular and organ sensations - recalled hunger, giant hives.

Stage 1b. Combined physio-verbal unit encoding - at height at two and a half years. - physiological encoding still occurs as verbal representations are added to encoded memory. The combined unit, thus produced, carries the sense of reality of its physiological component. Myths and explanations of experiences and events taught in words by caretakers carry this sense of reality into encoded memory. Whether as a result of fixation or regression, recall of these words are felt to be irrevocably real. Identity, political beliefs and religious dogma feel immutably real to the point that in defense of a concept, even war and the taking of life feels justified.

STAGE 1c. primary certainty- Concrete Verbal Encoding [encoding in shared words] -dominates from two to eight years. Words at first are linked to somatic memory elements without sensed boundaries, The participation in blended memory moieties (words and affects) of previously experienced internal sensations, transfers a narcissistic sense of certainty to the word contents representing memory and an unchalengeabilty to the concepts represented, Certainty is derived from the intuitive conclusion that repeatability verifies. Such certainty experience is called **primary certainty**.

Stage 2a The introduction of shared sustained awareness between a child and a caretaker maintained through shared words with mutually shared meanings creates a shared awareness.

Stage 2b Within this shared sustained awareness, there occurs at 24-30 Months, the introduction through displacement of weak symbols, whose transparency makes their meaning easy to discover. (i.e. phytophobia)

Stage 2c   Transparency is lost with the strengthening of repression that occurs at four years. The manifest symbol becomes a countercathexis element, which attracts awareness and makes the latent meaning unknowable (unbewusst, repressed, unconscious) Night fears, infantile zoo-phobias occur. (See Freud 1909"Little Hans")

Stage 2d   Strong repression occurs, as a result of which internal discharge through fantasy formation supports a neutral relationship with the world. Internalized expression of conflict at 6 years to 12 years enables delay of immediate response to stress, which makes a state of educability. calm and educability possible. This state is called the state of latency.

Stage 3   Abstract verbal encoding - encoding in memory as verbal abstraction starts at eight years. Full abstract function is reached by eleven years of age (tested through proverb interpretation)

Stage 4   [advanced special forms the poet, the artist the singer] 13 to 15 years and beyond.

STAGES ONE AND TWO OF ENCODING DISCUSSED

Stage 1 Physiological memory [preverbal]

Birth to Two Years

The first encodings, before there are words, are physiological sensations, which represent trauma. They can re-enter awareness as a regressed expression of a verbal recall. Examples of this process follow-

A. The hungry baby's hunger cries are stilled by the sound of mother coming.

B. A nineteen year old patient interrupted her associations to experienced abortions with the command "look". She simultaneously pointed to a giant hive that was rising on her forearm. I asked her **"What were you thinking just before this happened?"** Answered she, "I was thinking - 'I'd like to rip your guts out like they did mine." As she said this return to expression through words, the hive receded. Somatic memory elements provide a paradigm for regressive expression through psychosomatic symptoms. Fixation paradigms, which guide regressive activation of somatically encoded experience produces psychosomatic symptoms. Note: many psychosomatic symptoms reflect memory of haptically available and remembered events and perceptions effecting the body at the meeting of inside and outside. (mouth, lungs, rectum, integument).

Sensations and experiences are sources. When encoded they attract awareness (extended attention) as components of memory. Two types of such entities exist Those associated with affect, which serve as mnemic symbols of trauma, and those which are unaccompanied by physiological sensations (affect), such as numbers (acquired. during the phase of the acquisition of words). A splitting of extended awareness (Freud 1897 P 244) produces two entities, consciousness and unconsciousness. This splitting occurs during the somatic memory phase. Its exact time of occurring is less certain than its strengthening during the introduction of words as memory moieties.

The split produces three entities. The first are neutral numbers and their kin, which remain unnoticed and out of awareness until called upon by ambient needs. The second are memory entities, which are accompanied by discomforting affects. They push toward awareness like a sore thumb. Their presence in awareness could distract attention from survival and future planning. They are removed from awareness by expression of their meanings through displaced channels, such as activation of related somatic memory signs and symptoms, counter-cathexes, and symbols; all with less affect. This process truncates awareness; producing a reduced zone of extended attention awareness. The third entity consists of symbols and somatizations. These are displaced expressions of reminiscences that permit the entity to enter awareness in the form of sublimation, life patterns, and creativity (sublimation). Through these entities (reminiscences) expressed in play, dreams, and psychosomatic symptoms, abreaction and resolution of the disquieting content in the unconscious can be discharged or resolved.

Note: Consciousness is a physiological concept that describes wakefulness. It is a word, not an entity. Excluded from its definition is impaired awareness, such as "Anaesthetized", "Post Traumatic Coma", "Drug Overdose Coma", "Delta Wave Sleep" and "Deep Hibernation", Its use to represent "Truncated Attention Awareness", which is the product of psychological mechanisms of defense, 'poisons the well' from which the physiological understanding of "Consciousness" can be drawn.

Stage 2 Concrete verbal Encoding [encoding in words]

The introduction of words as memory moieties

By two and a half years of age the role of words in communicating and remembering becomes dependable. At first remembered words are linked with somatic memory elements without boundaries. The word, so joined, carries, as part of itself, affects based on the somatic memory elements. Percepts become memory contents, shaped from facets of the original percept mixed with traces of the affects (physiological feelings) experienced when the percept was first encountered. A metamorphic transformation occurs. Percepts are transformed into a cognitive memory mosaic. Two mosaic memory units can be identified falsely as being identical, based on a single shared facet. For example: Indians are swift. Antelopes are swift. Therefore antelopes are Indians. (THE MODE OF BARBARA). This is concrete thinking. Concrete Verbal Encoding reduces a percept to a preconception that fulfills personally driven hope. As "A single sparrow does not make a spring." (Aristotle 3rd century BC), so a shared single facet does not make an identity. Concrete thinking cannot be relied upon to establish reality. Such thinking is to be expected in children before the age of eight years.

Through precept and example during interaction with adults after eight years of age, percepts can become concepts, which can be identified as identical with other percepts, on the basis of a multitude of shared intrinsic factors. This is abstract thinking. There are societies that forbid such thinking (Munderocu). It is the basis for the scientific study and identification of reality.

Affect draws awareness to concepts. The affect-word concept entity encoded in memory therefore moves consistently toward awareness. If the concept is too uncomfortable, it is removed from access to sustained attention through displacement of its expression to less affect loaded entities such as symbols in play, dreams and fantasy.

At first, in early childhood, substitute entities (symbols) hold sustained attention weakly. For example, if a child of two and a half years of age presents with a seaweed phobia, a direct question such as "Who are you angry at?" will bring forth an answer such as "My mommy". This mild exclusion from awareness is called suppression.

Full attention, to the counter-cathected feared object, with exclusion from awareness of the entity defended against, is called repression. Repression first appears at four years of age, according to Piaget (1945). At. four years of age, strong repression produces infantile zoophobia.

PERCEPTUAL INFLUENCES ON MEMORY CONTENT.

A review of what is "encoded in memory "will be helpful in understanding the nature, limitations, and vulnerability of the of memories of patients in therapy. There are two types of perceptions that are encoded in memory. The first are Haptic perceptions, which include internal body experiences and near external events. These are detected through sensory receptors which are sensitive to immediate surroundings. The second are Telereceptor perceptions. which are acquired at a distance through hearing and sight.

HAPTIC

Internal sources encoded as haptic memory

Haptic memory, which contains encoded internal source sensations, is primarily involved in the interpretation and reflex response to the internal sensations which accompany life homeostasis and survival. These sources are encoded in memory through individual receptors or through a multitude of sensations which go to the brain for interpretation based on early learning.

The multiple internal sources encoded as haptic memory sensations consist of:

Tiredness

Anxiety

Parting, longing

Depression

Anger

Emunctory sensations [see Luria 1987]

EXTERNAL SOURCES ENCODED AS HAPTIC MEMORY

Heat

Being held

Skin contact

.Taste

Heat

Cold

Pain

Both internal and external sources make direct contribution to haptic memory through body based perceptual receptors.

Telereceptor Memory

External sources make direct input through perceptual receptors in the ear and eye. The experienced elements are often distant as in a landscape, or a concert or a conversation, or a lecture or a film. The encoded element, if recalled, does not have the intense sense of reality experienced while dreaming or remembering word-affect linked encodings (dogma) of phase 1b.

Telereceptor content acquired through the eyes and ears, such as landscapes and words become day residues and the facts of reality. They are stored in their own component of memory, from which they can be called for thinking with words and abstractions. Telereceptor sensations are also encoded as haptic content. Haptic memory therefore contains both encoded physiological experience, and telereceptor derived content, which are available to the dreaming brain.

Visual encoding / auditory encoding can be used for interpreting new experiences, or as a source of abstract encoded meaning to be applied during symbol formation. The encoded element serves as a paradigm for recognition or interpretation of new perceptions and experiences. Because telereceptor perception deals with items at a distance, and can be shared, it is majorly better than haptic impressions such as fantasies and wishes as sources for interpretation of shared scientific observations.

A REVIEW OF ENCODING AND THE SCIENTIFIC METHOD

Stage 1. PRENATAL THROUGH PREVERBAL physiological encoding involves feelings (Prenatal to 2 ½ years)

Regression to this stage produces psychosomatic signs.

Stage 2. Physiological/verbal encoding – (Strongest at 2 ½ to 4 yrs).

Words are encoded as compound entities made up of words and feelings. Depending on caretaker influence, new verbal endowments can be acquired indefinitely

Words reflecting endowed truths are encoded and retained in memory as a part of an insoluble entity made up of word phrases linked in memory to real physiological memory sensations. Through this linkage, words acquire a sense of reality. This is derived from the reality that was a real experience belonging to body function. Later remembered or recognized experiences expressed in words feel real. Acquisition of endowed memory for interpreting new experiences and sensation occurs when mythic word entities are used by caretakers to explain the world. "Endowed" truth is a term introduced by St. Thomas Aquinas to describe religious truths; told and heard.

Regression to this stage of encoding produces verbal recalls linked to a sense of reality –

STAGE 3 NEUTRAL VERBAL ENCODING BEGINS

With acquisition of words without affects.

As early as learning numbers. (about two years)

> When meanings for words are shared with
> others, personalized concepts give way
> to culturally defined entities.
> Then "EMOTIONAL BECOMES RATIONAL"
> and
> THROUGH SHARED VERBALIZATION
> "consensual validation"
> is introduced

The development of thought now faces gateways to two different pathways, by which to traverse life and its vicissitudes. One remains locked into a guidance derived from an endowed reality by which events are conceived and interpreted. The other pathway permits one to explore new understandings of reality, from which one can design a strategy to put the future into one's own hands, and cause the influence of fate to dwindle. Frankfort (1977) wrote of "the data of experience", as a forceful factor in the emancipation of thought from myth, produced when one learns to value consistency over probability. Then endowed knowledge, which belongs to the two dimensional world of the remembered written page gives way to the sway of the three dimensional world of verifiable, repeatable, and transmissible, remembered experience. This stripping off of "all the prescriptive sanctities of myth" clears the way for autonomy of thought. (p 386)

PSYCHOTHERAPEUTIC ASPECTS OF VARIATIONS OF ENCODINGS WITH AGE

An amalgam of maturation and tradition shape the form and boundaries of the ontogenetic progression described above. Psychotherapy can intrude on the products of this process.

Drawing a dream can access Haptic content for a therapist with children who have not yet reached the abstract capacity to get the main idea from a narrative or a dream and report it Endlessly detailed reports of dreaming occur especially in early latency. The drawing of the dream provides images of details which can be mounted as puppets, about which one can ask "Can you tell me about these figures?"

MEMORY, AGE, AND COGNITION

Vygotsky, (see Luria 1974) said in the early 1920's "Although a young child thinks by remembering, an adolescent remembers by thinking." (Page 11) The cognitive organizations which are involved in this change are named, in order of increasing maturation: affecto-motor memory organization, verbal conceptual memory organization, and abstract conceptual memory organization. These are the primary conduits through which the world of experience is apprehended and carried forward in time by memory. When one considers that the definition of consciousness that characterizes the theory of psychotherapy revolves about awareness of perception in the context of prior experiences of the perception and future implications of the perception, one must reach the conclusion that pathological turnings in the ways of memory are central to the understanding of pathological behavior and symptoms.

Affecto-Motor Memory Organization

The affecto-motor memory organization begins in life's first years. It consists of two components;

motor components and affective components. The
motor component is the first to be acquired. It
consists of purposefully modified patterns of motor
activity. Essentially, the contents of memory of this
component are syntaxes consisting of interrelating
motor components.

The affect component of the affecto-motor memory
organization is made up of the ability to evoke
recall of learned patterns in the form of affects,
perceptions, and bodily postures associated with an
initial experience. It represents the ability to
organize recall about sensory experiences. These
are usually recalled in their entirety.

Conceptual Memory

Conceptual memory is defined as the ability to
evoke recall of learned patterns in the form
of verbal signifiers such as words and related
symbols. Conceptual memory can be divided into the
earlier appearing verbal conceptual memory and
the relatively late appearing abstract conceptual
memory.

Verbal Conceptual Memory Organization

Verbal conceptual memory organization is able to be
operative by the third year of life at the latest.
It is not the primary means of memory used until
about six years of age. That is when latency begins.
The extent to which it is activated is determined
by environmental and social factors.

Abstract Conceptual Memory Organization

Abstract conceptual memory organization refers to a maturation based modification of conceptual memory. It appears first between seven and a half and eight and a half years of age. It consists of the skill of interpreting events in terms of their intrinsic nature and retaining the substance of this in memory through abstractions with or without words. (see also Sarnoff 1976 Pp 117-120 and 1987A Page 281 etseq.) The usual area of childhood activity in which such interpretation takes place is in "getting the main idea" in reporting dream and during reading. By the age of twelve accumulation of abstractions in memory should have reached the point at which abstractions can be applied to the interpretation of other abstractions. Children who fail to achieve this have trouble getting the main idea in reading, doing reports that require summaries of multiple sources, reporting dreams, and three part word problems in math.

COGNITIVE DEVELOPMENT AND PATHOLOGY

Though an adult who centers his life on fantastic evocations of his inner needs has lost his way, a child who treads the fantasy path is involved in acceptable behavior. Fantasy symbols serve the satisfaction of needs in the world of childhood where there are no handholds in reality to grasp for the fulfillment of inner wishes. A unique therapeutic approach must be developed to tap the world of the unbound energies and unbound wishes that are locked up in the symbols of the dreams, play and latent fantasies of the latency age child. Latent fantasies are the roots; manifest fantasies are the stalks and leaves; and dreams and play are the fruits and flowers in the wishing bowers from which the symptoms of neurosis also find expression and grow. Neurotic symptoms are formed when the manifest form of symbols, which represent these unconscious wishes, are pathologically reshaped by cognitive structures of the ego in service to the moral and ethical demands of the outside world.

Cognitive Pathologies Associated with
Disorders of Symbolic Thinking

Sir Henry Head (1920-1921), the early twentieth century British neurologist identified disordered symbolization as pathology. He described "... pathological repression that causes all sorts of distorted personal symbols to encroach on literal thought and empirical judgment and abstract concepts..." to be an abrogation of human freedom. Loss of "...imagination to envisage our problems clearly and negotiably..." block free functioning of mind. He felt that "... the most disastrous hindrance is disorientation, the failure or destruction of life-symbols..." (P 290), which explain the unknown, orient one within the world, and harness awareness for future use through encoding the symbols of awareness into abstract memory.

Head divides the symbolizing function into two aspects. First there are afferent processes, which through creating reduced representations, make possible the codification of experiences in memory for use as referent concepts. Second there are efferent processes that select symbols for the manifest expression of referent concepts. Impaired afferent symbolization occurs when there is an inability to create abstractions as a result of impaired ability to recognize and reorganize similarities. Impaired efferent symbolization is seen when ability to find a way to expression is hobbled by limitation of symbolic linkages to concrete similarities, or by displacements too diffuse to give form to expressions. Such an impaired displacement during symbolization occurs when there is absence of high level abstraction applied through symbolic linkages during efferent symbolic expression. Such a loss occurs in aphasias (See Head (1920-1921) – and in the regressed symbolizations based on concrete superficial similarities that occur in dreams, neuroses, psychoses, direct discharge into autonomic expression, and the concrete thinking of the early (before eight years old) latency age child.

Clearly there is more to the role of "attending to symbols" during psychotherapy, than the interpretation of latent meanings that were derived from stressful situations confronting the patient. The process of symbol formation should also be addressed. Head (1920-1921) offered insight into the goals of this aspect of therapy. He noted that "in order that words can sub-serve intellectual activity, they must be mobilized and capable of manipulation at will." (P 180) and "Want of perfect recognition of verbal significance leads to a defective power of naming." (P193) Encouragement of fantasy and learning to manipulation referents through displacement (encouraging fantasy through improved symbolization) becomes an important element in psychotherapeutic endeavors with children.

NEUROSES OF CHILDHOOD

The neuroses of the young come into being as a compromise between unconscious longings and the unbending demands of reality. Longings rise toward consciousness from zones where energies are free to seek discharge without the restraint of object, place, time or accidents of fate. There, free energies run the errands of desire in fantasy filled pleasure palaces of the mind. When free energies are confronted with those stringent demands of reality that bind them to obligations, their pathways to expression become limited. Locked to the harsh realities of the world, where oncoming adult size and knowledge acquisition impinge on the free small world of the humble child, they become bound energies. The older the child, the weaker is the influence of childish wishes and the stronger the influence of reality. Between the two extremes lie zones, of hope and fantasy tinted compromise, from which the neuroses of the young arise.

The neuroses of prelatency, latency, and early adolescence differ from adult neuroses in the degree to which they are influenced by maturation. With the exception of the intensification of obsessional defenses in the late twenties, the matrix of adult cognition that gives rise to neurosis is relatively fixed. By comparison, the underpinnings of neurosis in the young are in constant maturational flux, and there is an ebb and flow of drive energies and of external pressures. One of the clinical products of this is the transient nature of symptoms in the young neurotic.

Latent fantasy contents change in response to new siblings, humiliations, school challenges and vicissitudes of parental adjustment beyond the control of the child. Rarely is the childhood neurosis an organizer that by its very existence holds its finger in a dike to counter inner pressures and permit the remaining ego some degree of autonomy, creating neutral ego functioning in the service of adaptation as adult neuroses and perversions sometimes do.

Childhood neurosis is evidence of a weak spot, whose presence is pervasively disorganizing. The child therapist must be tuned in for many more factors than the adult therapist. He must be ever on the alert for alteration in the potential for neurotic symptom formation that is introduced by normal cognitive maturation, and persistent immaturities that spring into action when maturation fails to keep pace with the passing years. Childhood neurosis is like a volcanic island that grows by rising from the sea under pressure from afar, all the while adding to its bulk by eruptions. It has many sources for its features. The child therapist must be familiar with the sources of childhood neurosis, both the ebb

and flow of life's tides and the somewhat eldritch
isostacy engendered by cognitive transformations.

The neutral world of the child, supported by bound
energies, can be approached through verbal exchanges
in therapy sessions. This touches only the civilized
crust of a child's existence. There are more personal
zones of life. Drive derivatives do not gain easy
entrance to reality interactions. Discharge of the
drives is buffered by a recreation of the world
through displacement of its elements into symbolic
forms. Adjustment in large part revolves about the
maintenance of a symbol-based world of fantasy.

DREAMS AND PLAY IN THE TREATMENT OF NEUROSIS IN THE YOUNG

Cognition, manifest symbols and fantasy, are
the building blocks from which the elements of
unconscious mental life such as latent fantasy
can be shaped into conscious representations.
Latent fantasy can be held in memory for extended
periods of time, making it possible to transport
early life experience to the present, whence it
can influence normal and pathological manifest
forms of behavior. Normal behavior includes dreams,
play, and transference. Aberrant behavior includes
symptoms and characerological behavior. The fantasy
antecedents of aberrant behavior and of play, dreams,
and transference are shared. A key to understanding
characterological pathology and symptoms should be
discoverable in the latent fantasies, which share
by both healthy and pathological derivatives. Latent

fantasy can be discerned in the stories and symbols
of play and dreams.

Both cognition and fantasy can produce pathology.
Aberrations in cognitive function create aberrant
behavioral forms. Cognitive function influences
the choice of current manifestation of fantasy
from among such possibilities as symptoms, play,
dreams, or behavior. Latent fantasy contributes
to its content. Therapy of children should be
geared to the treatment of pathological content
as well as the pathological form taken by the
psychopathology of childhood. The goal of therapy
in dealing with the neuroses of the young is to
relieve psychopatho-genetic current distress while
enhancing the natural growth of the personality.
The therapist attempts to move the child towards
an ability to test reality so well that his adult
life will not be lived far removed from fact; and
he will be able to deal with reality directly rather
than through misinterpreting it.

To understand the manifestations of the unconscious
as they impact on the psychotherapeutic situation
in the young, the development of that aspect of
cognition (symbol formation, fantasizing function,
and cognition function) that reworks content into
cryptic forms must be at the therapist's finger tips.
There is no time to 'look it up', while conducting
psychotherapy sessions. This knowledge offers a basis
for identifying change in behavior, symbol, fantasy
or symptom that has been produced by interpretation.
Such gain should be differentiated from changes
that are the result of maturation of cognitive

function. This differentiation provides guidelines
for increasing therapeutic emphasis, when needed,
in the direction of altering cognition and enhancing
reality testing rather than interpretation of the
content of latent fantasy in the psychotherapy of
the latency and late-latency-early adolescent child.

DREAM INTERPRETATION

Dream symbols, by their nature provide far less
entré for the therapist than ludic symbols. Dream
symbols are limited. They can be studied for clues to
meaning in a dream. They cannot be selected freely,
introduced by the therapist, colored, exchanged,
or altered by a conscious wish. They have fixed
initial alterations in form made necessary by the
primarily visual character of their source. There is
therapeutic potential in turning dream symbols into
ludic symbols by making them into cutout puppets.

Playroom toys can be added to play therapy by a
therapist as ludic symbols. They can be adapted to
serve all the whim driven ways of human desiring.
Past hurts and failures can be relived through them
and strong self images restored.

Dream symbols are primarily visual and less
malleable. This is not psychologically determined.
This is the effect of biochemical processes on the
organization of memory. Dreams are seen, because
the stuff of dreams is drawn from memory areas that
are limited in what they hold; telereceptor visual
imagery. Distortion in representation is inherent
in the process of using symbolic forms that are

limited to visual forms. Interpretation of dream symbols requires conclusions removed from the hope and fear, wish and fulfillment that is the stuff of dream longing. Confirmation of interpretive conclusions depends on further associations.

JDS

What is the stuff that dreams are made of?

CAS

Dreams are made up of self awareness and hope expressed in visually coded situations. Visual encoding is usual in dreams but is not necessary. People, born blind, dream. Mrs. Dorothy Birmingham (1962), of the Hampstead Clinic in London, presented a dream of a blind child. Not a trace of visual imagery was present in the dream. The child reported that in the dream she was descending the stairs. She prepared to turn right into the living room, where her mother was. She knew her mother was down and to the right, because that was the direction that she sensed in the dream from which her mother's perfume was coming.

During REM dreaming the mind is isolated from objects in reality. Its use of symbols resembles that of the latency age child who plays with ludic symbols in the absence of the availability of physiologically based personality structures that would enable him to articulate drives with real objects in real situations. The marked attenuation of the influence of supplies of reality sensation during REM is a result of a physiological blocking of the influence of external visual input. This blocking is caused by two forces.

The **first** is rapid movement of the retina during REM. During eye movement no retinal input to the brain is recognized. This phenomenon is associated with all eye movement. It can be demonstrated while awake simply by looking at a mirror while shifting one's gaze from the right pupil to the left pupil. One cannot see the movement. This scientific physiological finding was described by Pompeianu in 1970. He reported that there is no neural transmission from the retina to the visual cortex in REM sleep (page 10). Pompeianu's findings could explain de-emphasis of reality-based visual influence on symbol formation during REM dreaming.

The **second** is a biochemically based alteration in the organization of sources of recall for dreams. For instance, during REM sleep production of noradrenaline in the locus coeruleus stops and the effect of serotonin neurons is silenced while acetylcholine neurons remain very active. Dominance of acetylcholine in the brain produces a shift in the cognitive content available to awareness. There is a decrease in brain activity in the dorsolateral prefrontal cortex and an increase in brain activity in the region of the visual cortex. The REM state associated shift from catecholeamine frontal lobe dominance to acetylcholine occipital lobe dominance could explain the predominance of visual imagery based symbols and the altered nature of symbolization in REM sleep. There is blockage of inputs derived from the prefrontal cortex and the external organs of perception, including perceptions encoded as abstractions, and verbal forms derived from visually encoded memories. Physostigmine in the brain enhances brain activity in the region of the visual cortex. (see Sarnoff (2002) vol 1, p 260) This increases the visual content available for dream symbols. That could be why visual images dominate in dreams.

As a result of de-emphasis of external visual inputs, REM dream symbols become primarily the products of haptic internal visual evocations. Other modalities such as hearing and smell, remaining under the muting influence of reality are preempted. As a result an unleashed intensely visual evocative mode dominates REM dream content. For this reason, REM dream symbols are primarily visual with sources, which are internal and evocative.

Haptic sensations that propel these symbols are experienced as anxiety. The anxiety affect associated with evocative symbols represents the energy of drives that stand ever at the ready to propel internal conflict into conscious awareness.

BRAIN CHEMISTRY AND DREAMING

SUMMARY

There is predominance, of acetylcholine and a cessation of catecholamine activity in the brain during REM sleep. This results in a dorsolateral prefrontal brain activity decrease with a shift to the visual memory area of the occipital lobe as a source of manifest dream symbols. Since during REM sleep external visual stimuli are blocked durin movement of the retina, the dream symbols of the REM state are entirely derived from occipital lobe haptic visual memories. During manifest dream symbol formation, displacement from affect filled latent content to manifest REM dream symbols occurs; laden with less affect. Second stage EEG dreaming is therefore normally calm and pictorial.

Blocking of external sensations excludes reality sources from dream awareness. Chemical changes of EEG second stage REM states, strengthen the contribution of the occipital lobe visual memory area to dreaming awareness. As a result manifest dream symbols are visual. Defensive displacement during transformation to manifest dream content from latent content reduces affect. Transformation of occipital lobe latent content into calm visual manifest dream symbols in dream awareness, through displacement and neutralization, supports the persistence of sleep.

THE LATENCY PERIOD

The Latency period is the time period from 6 yrs to 12 yrs during which "the structure of latency", (an organization of defenses) can produce the calm, quiet, and educability that permits effective learning in school. The name was suggested to Freud by a colleague (W. Fleiss) to identify the period in childhood from which, during adult analyses memories are not produced spontaneously during free association. The memories remain latent.

Use of the single word, "latency" conjures up the workings of the secret world of childhood. Other words have been used to describe this period. They require extensive modifiers to limit the extent of the time period under study. For instance "the school years" are understood to represent preschool, kindergarten, grade school, high school, and college. An added demurrer is required to establish new limits. "The middle child" has an established meaning. It refers to the child born between the youngest child and the oldest child, When there are three siblings, the term is appropriate from infancy through senility. An added demurrer is required to establish new limits. (For more information on "Latency", see Sarnoff (1976))

Latency is not a silent time during which to wait for adolescence, nor is it an adventitious element cast into the great sea of development. Latency is more than a moment that leaves a little mark in passing. All of development must flow through the Structures of Latency, which produce states of latency. (see Sarnoff (1976)) Adolescence evolves out of the cognitive transitions of latency. Psychotherapy for adolescents must be informed by knowledge of that which can go wrong during the transitions that precede it. Psychotherapy during the latency years therefore affects not only immediate emotional problems, but also the long range effects of distortions that occur during latency age development. From the standpoint of pathological development, the aspects of latency and adolescence that are most sensitive and most often in need of help are those functions that take part in finding comfort in fantasy, maturation of object relations, the transformations in cognition that enhance reality testing.

The existence of the "structure of latency" was brought into focus for me in stunning fashion. The father of a patient called for an appointment to see me. His son was a rebellious late latency child who often fought with his father at the dinner table. The father came with advice to give me, rather than in search of information. He advised me to augment my techniques with foolproof advice for parents; aimed at bringing wayward youngsters into line. I

listened eagerly in hope of getting good advice.
"Beat them!" said the father, "That's what I do.
When he doesn't behave at the table, I beat him. He
runs away bawling, but is back in a few minutes as
quiet and well behaved as you could want." I could
not convince the father of the error of his ways. He
was sure of his technique because the results were
so good. In the next session with the boy, when I
asked him about the effect of beating a child, he
confided that it worked well. "At first I'm angry."
said he. "I run upstairs saying, 'I could kill him.
I could kill him.' I throw myself on the bed and
shout it into my pillow. Then it's all gone. I feel
okay. I go back downstairs. I eat. Everything is
calm. You should tell the other parents about it."
He had been doodling as he talked. I Asked him to
explain what appeared to be a map. "It's the banks
near here," said he, "I'm planning a robbery." He
unfolded a fantasy of robbing banks, his parents,
and his neighbors. One of his presenting complaints
was robbing a drug-store. The reaction to the
beating by his father had been dissipated through
the medium of fantasy. Real objects are not sought
for the discharge of drives during latency as
they are during early childhood and adolescence.
Fantasy containing ludic symbols (see Unit Five
below) becomes the channel for discharge. When
real objects are involved, they serve as armatures
upon which form derived from fantasy is projected.
When a latency age child is stressed, a pattern
of pathways for discharge is activated. Drives and
feelings involved in the response to stress are
dissipated through fantasy.

I soon found that this dissipation of stress response was not the only process that resolved stress through verbal fantasy pathways for discharge. The normal excitements, seen for instance in pre-latency children, which had been discharged through masturbation, contact with objects, and evocation of memories of past experiences of gratification, are denied expression for long periods by teachers and parents of latency age children. Participation in culture myths are provided as alternatives for use in discharging energies. In this way, drives are harnessed to the process of acquiring the traditions of a culture.

I came to call this pattern of pathways for discharge, which operates when other pathways are blocked or forbidden, the *structure of latency*. When this process is active, available, and effective, the latency age child is in a *state of latency*. It is the potential for achieving this state that defines the years six to twelve as the latency period.

Fantasy in Latency

Latency is a magic road that wends its way through a landscape of fantasies. Of these fantasies, derivatives of the oedipus complex loom like mountain ranges. Tracing the same course, but as foothills, are anal-sadistic preoccupations. Scattered along the way, as the latency years unfold, there is a march of fantasy responses to the challenges that accompany cognitive, physical, and social maturation. The challenges include humiliation, sibling rivalry, budding sexuality, and passivity.

LATENCY AND FANTASY

There are two directions that dynamic psychotherapy of children can take. One entails encouraging the maturation of cognition, especially in the areas of reality testing and the types of objects from which the symbolic forms of manifest fantasy are derived. The second entails resolution of latent fantasy and discharge of drives and tension through the encouragement by the therapist of working through and cathartic abreaction with memory alteration that results when fantasy play uses ludic symbol containing fantasy.

It is natural and an occupier of much time for the child to engage in fantasy and fantasy play during waking life. It is as natural to fantasy while awake, as it is for all ages to dream at night. In the child therapy session, it is possible to tap this process and adapt it to therapeutic growth, resulting in discharge of drives, resolution of fantasy contents, and encouragement of cognitive growth, freeing the child to enter adulthood unencumbered.

Technically tapping this process refers to intervention by the therapist, in which ludic symbols are introduced through the early ludic portal. Suggestion, dream element emphasis, drawing, puppet play, and interpretive clay modeling are used. (see "therapeutic entry points", and "the ludic portal" in the "circle of change" in "Roy, The Boy Who Would be King" in UNIT V below.)

The Age Frames of Fantasy

The Stage of Early Latency

Oedipality and Guilt

At the beginning of the latency period, before attendance at grade school begins (five to six years of age), pleasing fantasy content is informed by the oedipus complex. As the child reaches six, the capacity to experience guilt develops. Then oedipal fantasies (taking the roles of either of the parents) cease to be the sources of pleasant musings. Associated with guilt, their potential entry into consciousness generates fear. and expected retribution. These responses are transmuted into manifest fantasies of theft and imprisonment. Such fantasies discharge tension. In a part of the psyche, sequestered from reality, they provide a sense of expiation or mastery for the feelings and situations involved. Such fantasies dominate the latency age period.

Should these fantasies fail to resolve oedipal pressures, tne ego responds with a regression that directs attention to anal sadistic preoccupations, replacing the newer and more perilous oedipus complex with an area which has already been dealt with in prior years – now to be confronted with a far more sophisticated and mature set of defenses. In the healthiest possible response, the anal sadistic impulses are defended against by the mobilization of the "MECHANISMS OF RESTRAINT" (reaction formation, symbolization, isolation, doing and undoing, and obsessive compulsive defenses) which defuse the strength of the drives that impel the child to fantasy. The mechanisms of restraint produce a STATE OF LATENCY in the child to the casual observer appears to have socially appropriate periods of calm, pliability, reasonableness and educability. These attributes underlie readiness for the activities of the grade and junior high school years.

Should drives be stirred by maturation or accidents of fate (physical and sexual growth, losses, sexual exposure, seduction, humiliation and beatings), there is a danger that stress will be placed beyond the control of the mechanisms of restraint and the state of calm be lost. This alternative is averted by the assertion of an organization of the ego with an unique association to latency. This is "THE STRUCTURE OF LATENCY" (See above and Sarnoff 1976 pages 13-36) which serves as a safety valve to preserve the state of latency. This is an ego configuration that provides alternative outlets for excess drive energies. By deflecting drive energies and diminishing the pressure on the static and brittle mechanisms of restraint, it becomes a support for a successful defensive against regression to anal sadistic preoccupations, and clears the decks of any need for conscious attention to oedipal concerns. The action of the structure of latency, excludes the offending stress from consciousness; its content is fragmented, then displaced, and then represented by symbols which are organized into manifest fantasies which become the dreams, play, and daydream fantasies of childhood. Often the child, unequipped to deal with the dragons of reality, turns to victories in these fantasies as recompense and resolution for the problems of the day. In this way anal sadistic preoccupations are defeated by the structure of latency.

They are never totally vanquished. Within cohorts of peers cloistered in the permissive zone found in the backseats of carpool vehicles, they sing of "dooty" and of a man, with diarrhea. (see the movie "Parenthood"). To avoid disorganizing play in therapy sessions, don't interpret or try to alter the structure of latency.

With the passing of years, additional fantasy contents appear, resulting in a de-emphasis of Oedipal fantasy in the middle and late latency years. These contents are responses to the problems presented to the child during the stage of latency age development at which they occur.

The Stage of Middle Latency

A sense of independence from parents at about seven or eight years of age, projects a child into a psychic reality, marked by separation and loneliness feelings, in which he is all alone in the big world. Fear fantasies of being small, and vulnerable follow. The impotence felt may be symbolized by a dread of monsters, which represent both what they fear and serve as masking vehicles for projections of the child's own defensively mobilized aggression.

The Stage of Late Latency

Passivity

Beyond the age of nine or ten, the problem of passivity becomes a major issue. A sense of independence develops at this age, which reaches a point at which children strongly wish to break free of parental control. They object to the passive role that they have to take in relation to the decision making parent. This is in many ways a recapitulation of the two year old demand to know, "Who's the boss of me". These children would like to run their own lives. They object to parental control and interference on an ever widening horizon of activities. Eventually this trend becomes so intense that they have little else on their minds. The child confronts the parent with "Don't treat me like a baby!" This is evidence of a child readying himself to turn his adaptive energies, from inward turning fantasies which solve problems through the manipulation of symbols, to demands and actions that will intrude on the world. The children become especially sensitive to situations in which their decisions are challenged or their immaturity emphasized.

The Stage of Late Late Latency

Ethical Individuation

Sensitivity to challenge to the child's social decisions leads to feelings of humiliation and inferiority, when ethical conflicts estrange them from their parents. This can include simple choices such as crossing the street alone or major decisions in response to peer pressure involving stealing, drugs and sex. In defense, the children generate fantasies about being movie stars, championship athletes, owning motorbikes, etc. Some children who are conflicted about such confrontations deflect the challenge into fantasies of defiance. These can take the form of fantasies of theft and crime which are at times acted out.

The Stage of Late Latency - Early Adolescence

Sexual Identity Crises

Awakening concern about sexual identity intensifies with the first growth spurt. This occurs at about nine years of age. Body changes, though too slight to be detected by a casual observer, alert the child to pubertal changes. Children revive old concerns about sexual identity. They worry about what they'll look like as adults. It is not uncommon for boys to mistake breast buds as evidence of a sex change. This stirs up other fantasies and castration fears.

During late latency, size and hormones and available reality partners make fantasy as defense less necessary. Reality offers satisfaction. The child grows, and ludic symbols dwindle. The cycle of change of the ludic symbol in latency comes to an end. A transition from thinking of objects in fantasy to seeking reality objects through future planning becomes a center of activity. This is ludic demise. The therapist is there to discuss and work through the child's hopes. The end of the cycle offers the therapist a portal of entry into the growing personality of the child. As during the beginning of the cycle the therapist can introduce elements from the ambient word to the child's choices during his establishment of his expectation driven interchange with reality. The therapist's intervention may be concrete or abstract depending on the child's level of cognition.

(see "therapeutic entry points" in the "circle of change" in "Roy, The Boy Who Would be King" in UNIT V below.)

The Vicissitudes of the Instincts Over time

In the Normal and Schizophrenic Child

There is a developmental line for object relations. In normal children, It starts with total narcissism in the first year of life and ends with the capacity to fall in love at about 15 years. Its stages are often linked to biological growth markers such as puberty. The validity of theories of connection to maturational events varies from positing to possible. There are three schizophrenia related diagnostic entities recognized in childhood; prepubescent schizophrenia, childhood schizophrenia, (and adult schizophrenia of early onset). Each entity has persistent autism as a symptom. By studying the vicissitudes of the instincts that determine their symptomatology at about twelve years of age (their typical age of appearance) their aberrant object relations pathology can be explored.

THE INSTINCTUAL PROFILE OF THE NORMAL CHILD
THROUGH THE YEARS

The phenomena that moves the normal child out of latency into adolescence is part of a race survival mechanism. (Freud 1915 p 126) There is a hormone driven shift from self evocation to reproductive creativity, requiring a procreation possible (nubile) real world object. The associated shift of instinctual cathexes from inside to outside goals and from evocation of self to communication with peers is a cognitive characteristic of the normal prepubertal period. During normal maturation there is a heightening of the power of reality to attract cathexes, and strengthen memory contents capacity to evaluate reality without fantasy elaboration. There is a shift from the use of evocative forms to communicative symbolic forms that is intensified in the normal child. A shift from evocative to communicative symbolic forms is intensified in the normal child by twelve years of age.

schizophrenic maturation

In schizophrenic maturation, each of the types of schizophrenia follows its own developmental course. For example, The shift of attention cathexes to reality involved in the childhood schizophrenic differs from the prepubertal schizophrenic's in that it is stronger, and is subject to regression to concrete operations and concrete verbal memory systems, while the prepubescent schizophrenic child regresses to the use of the affecto-motor memory system for clues to the interpretation of reality.

Regression from the abstractions needed for middle school tests to dependence on personalized affecto-motor memory based mythology provides mythic explanations for physical feelings. Cognitive style shifts can best be understood through study of changes in instinctual expression during the stages of maturation.

Freud (1915) delineated the characteristics by which instinctual expression can be described.

The characteristics are source, pressure, aim and object.

PROFILE OF THE NORMAL CHILD

The vicissitudes of the drive that impels love object seeking in normal development are

Source - Stimulus -→ need → satisfaction (page 119)

Internal Tissues
Hormones

Pressure - Demand for expression - heightened by increased release of sexual Hormone with start of puberty.

AIM - goal Discharge-→ pleasure → reproduction (p 126)

Aim is variable. (Page 122)

OBJECT - sought changes with cognitive growth over time, starting with one's own body as object (Page 122), and ending with an external love object.

The choice of object depends on the successive stages of maturational potential. These are:

Primary narcissism (P 136) -self

The Structure of Latency -regression and displacement away From objects toward symbols.

Reversal at 8 ½ -Shift from accommodation to self to assimilation to the world of interpretation and concepts Pubertal (hormonal) push toward an external object.

Capacity to fall in love at 15 years of age.

Some of the primary factors in differential diagnosis concern the nature and developmental history of the introject (internalized object) utilized in the formation of the feared persecutors. During the early latency age period, childhood schizophrenics tend to relate to internalized objects in the form of consciously fantasized little people or objects within their body boundaries. Children in more normal states relate to parents, peers of the same sex, and external objects in fantasy, which are not felt to be inside themselves. In nonpsychotic children who have internalized fantasy objects, the fantasy objects are patterned after actual experiences. They are derived from reality and external objects. Rapoport (1944), in comparing the relations of schizophrenic and normal children to internalized objects, stated: "As we turned from the psychoses and approached the neuroses, we found instead of the bizarre primitive and unrealistic fantasy objects [internalized objects] of the former, fantasy objects which were more conditioned by actual experiences and which were more related to reality and the external parents" (p. 320).

THE INSTINCTUAL PROFILE OF THE PREPUBESCENT SCHIZOPHRENIC CHILD AT TWELVE

Source Stimulus -→ need → satisfaction (page 119) Stimulus from Internal Tissues.

Pressure Increased demand for expression as sexual hormones increase with puberty

AIM   Discharge
self expressive evocations
self oriented communications.
There may be regression from functioning with neutral energies
to discharge-→ pleasure

OBJECT   First primary narcissism (P 136) seeks one's own body as object (Page 122)..
Verbal skills encourage contact with objects .
Accommodation of objects to self ideas and needs.
The Structure of Latency creates a regression and displacement away from objects toward symbols.
Reversal at 8 ½ Shift to assimilative (reality oriented)
Interpretation.
Pubertal (hormonal) push toward an external object.

From the therapeutic point of view, these findings
will help one to identify patients who will
not benefit from transference oriented dynamic
psychotherapies.

UNIT FOUR

THE MECHANISMS AND TECHNIQUE OF THERAPY

SYMBOLS MARK THE PLACE WHERE MEMORY OF HUMILIATION AND FAILURE, WITH THEIR AFFECTS, LIE IN WAIT; LONGING TO FIND EXPRESSION, SOMETIMES FINDING RESOLUTION.

THE MECHANISMS OF FANTASY

The fantasies produced by the structure of latency are highly symbolized, defensively constructed manifest fantasies. They are played out through the symbols of latency fantasy play. They mask latent fantasies. Latent fantasies are not just passive unconscious symbol patterns, awaiting a cue to come forth and take shape in the manifest fantasies of play. They are part of an active system of psychical forces, which are ever at the ready to bring prior events, expectations, unresolved experiences and traumas from the child's past into action in the interpretation and reaction of the child to new experiences and perceptions. An example of a pre-informed expectation is illustrated by the following experience of a prelatency youngster who was visiting his aunt. He asked for a cookie. There was no cookie in sight. The aunt improvised with the offer of a Rye-Krisp. The child took it, bit at it, and finding that it did not give way to his teeth as a proper cookie should, announced as he handed it back - "Aunt Carole, it doesn't work."

A child whose latent fantasies are influenced by sexual feelings for his parents will be apt to be stirred by seductive behavior to the point that the structure of latency (See Sarnoff 1976) will defensively produce an oedipal fantasy derivative in play. Failing this, there may be a shift in a regressive direction requiring the further mobilization of the mechanisms of restraint. The mechanisms of restraint deal primarily with regressions from oedipal fantasies. The latency defense of the structure of latency is less specific, since it is often called upon to deal with a multitude of possible complexes, sensitivities and instigators of anger, overwhelming excitements, humiliations and the many putdowns to which the psyches of our patients as children are prone.

The role of fantasy in the psychological life of the child extends much beyond serving as a place to hide from reality and feelings. Fantasy also helps to preserve family intactness. Fantasies can be used to discharge affects and tension. Manifest fantasy can be used to discharge, master, and resolve latent fantasies (referents) that serve as memory moieties which carry into latency traumas and conflicts of infancy and the prelatency period that if unresolved, threaten later life adjustment.

Fantasy and the Illusion of Knowledge

Anger at parents can be blunted by a change of topic in the child's mind's eye. This is an example of self distraction through fantasy. By substituting a symbol for a momentarily hated object, the child can produce a shift of cathexes (attention energy) from an emotionally uncomfortable area of contemplation to a more neutral one. The ego mechanism involved is called displacement. As a result of this phenomenon, the child produces for himself a life image that is shorn of painful reflections on the truth of the matter. A countercathectic "illusion of knowledge" (see Boorstin 1983 P86) pervades memory supporting the myth of an idealized family relationship. One is reminded of the biblical proverb that tells of the stratagem of focusing on a fantasy of a dangerous beast in order to avoid admitting to a disinclination to work or progress. ["The slothful man saith, There is a lion in the way; a lion is in the streets. (proverbs 6.13)]

Future Planning

When those whose fantasies are the product of an intact "Structure of Latency" reach adolescence, their capacity for future planning is strong. Early and middle latency fantasies are plans that bypass problems through distraction, drive discharge, and diminution of affect and mood. This is done through displacement from affect charged latent symbols to manifest symbols that carry or attract less affect. The manifest symbols of early latency are selected from non-human unrealistic elements which exist in a context of timelessness. As cognition matures bringing latency to its end, there is a shift in the symbolic forms from which manifest forms are selected. Late latency manifest symbols include real people in real situations in a linear time frame. With this change in symbols, the structure of latency has the potential to convert from a static structure to a personality skill. The latter solves reality problems through the creation of fantasies that plan for the future through the manipulation of the realities of the world. Thus does problem resolution evolve from alloplastic fantasy formation to autoplastic future planning. Enhanced reality testing runs parallel to this process. The more reality influenced are the symbols used in fantasy, and the more that symbols give way to real creatures in the daydreams of the young, the greater is the chance that the daydreams and play fantasies of childhood will be gratified through their new role as patterns and as guides to fulfillment in shaping adult life. This insight was acutely perceived by Rabindranath Tagore (1936) in his poem "The Beginning"

"Where have I come from, where did you pick me up?" the baby asks its mother.

She answered, half crying, half laughing, and clasping the baby to her breast. 'You were hidden in my heart as its desire, my darling. You were in the dolls of my childhood's games..." (page 14).

As the symbols of fantasy come to be drawn more and more from reality elements as their source, parents become involved in social interactions instigated by the child. The parental style of response provides for the child the patterns with which he will interact and encounter peers after removal of parents as primary love objects.

A therapy can intervene through offering insight into this process in two ways. Advice to parents can alter this influence on later social interaction.

A non-sadomasochistic relationship within the therapeutic situation can enhance the alternatives available for mature social interaction for the child.

Fantasy as Reparative Mastery

Ordinary daily events, when interpreted in the light of the charged memories that they call forth, can generate distortions of reality and misunderstandings. Such sources of tension can be reduced in a child by the defusing of such memories through discharge through fantasy dominated play of affects linked to them. Rage released in a fantasy locale reduces tension in reality venues such as home, school and arenas for play. Affects can be neutralized by displacement of activities to zones of calm where mastery can be assured.

Events generate conflict. Conflict can seek out events. The forces of mastery and repetition seek successful new experiences in reality to serve the same purpose as the generation of manifest fantasies, which heal through discharge, reassurance, and the resolution of past traumas. As a result, latent fantasies, which carry old imbalances in drive pressures into contemporary situations, are reduced. Cognitive transformations, which were slowed by distractions and anxiety, can then progress.

Fantasy as a Manifestation of Compulsion to Repeat

Persecutory fantasy, which in latency creates a cruel monster attacking the child, presages recurrent experiences of being treated cruelly by peers and lovers in later life, when real people are recruited to populate fantasies. Manifest fantasy content is synthesized from age appropriate symbolic forms associated with levels of development reached as the result of the cognitive transformations of latency. Repetition, in fantasy and reality, which fails to resolve the conflicts associated with underlying latent fantasy, are manifestations of repetition compulsion. Repetition in fantasy and reality, which resolve the conflicts associated with latent fantasy by successfully reliving and redoing the outcome of the original traumatic experience in the child's favor, are manifestations of reparative mastery.

The distinct nature of child and early adolescent psychotherapy is mandated by three pathological elements. These are: failure of fantasy or behavior to relieve instinctual pressures (repetition compulsion), failure to progress to age appropriate symbolic forms, and interference with object relations on a reality level by instinctual pressures that seek expression of fantasy through the manipulative use of real objects. Psychotherapeutic strategies in the treatment of neurosis in the young require techniques that attend to these problem areas. To be able to do this, the therapist must have an understanding of the disorders of age appropriate cognitive transformation which produce such pathologies.

(See above "The Neuroses of Childhood")

THE ROLE OF FANTASY IN THERAPY AND ADJUSTMENT

Encouragement of fantasy during psychotherapy enhances the effectiveness of an important developmental task of latency. This is the resolution and defusing of the impact of persistent memory referents based on trauma that occurred during pre-latency. Fantasy play makes its contribution to this process by giving the child a chance to discharge tension and master trauma through catharsis, by successfully reliving the past in thought. Fantasy in the growing child is normally manifested in thought and in words, in dreams and in play. In large measure, psychotherapy of the young adapts such normal fantasy activity to the goals of therapy. For the fantasy rich child, this is done through encouraging already present skills of fantasy play. For the child poor in capacity for the formation of fantasy and symbol, one attempts to enhance basic skills in the use of words and symbols. (See below "The Boy Who Would Be King") Fantasy as part of therapy serves as a medium for the discharge of tension. Tension discharge through fantasy can be achieved without interventions or interpretations by the therapist. Fantasy play can be used for mastery of current trauma as well.

Dynamic interpretation can harness fantasy play to therapeutic goals on a more complex level.

Usually in late latency abstract discussions of the
relationship between past traumas, manifest fantasy,
and symbol content can bring the relationship
of latent conflicts and their manifest fantasies
into awareness. This enhances the effectiveness
of psychotherapy by making unconscious content
available for discussion and as the starting
point for new associations. In this way, impact of
past and current traumas can be defused through
confrontation with reality.

Fantasy during latency contributes to adjustment in
later years. It serves as a proving ground for the
role of trial action (thought) in solving problems.
As the symbolizing function matures, reality objects
serve as sources of the symbol content of fantasies.
This enhances the application of reality testing in
judging the appropriateness of efforts at problem
solving. In this way, the trial action that is
implied in thought and fantasy grows to be future
planning. Failure of this natural developmental
step during latency produces an individual who
thinks in an egocentric non-linear manner, as seen
in amotivational syndromes and adolescent drug
users. (see Pittell (1973)

There are two kinds of experience that can encourage
this developmental shortfall. The first is severe
trauma that shatters the effectiveness of the
structure of latency. The second is the presence in
reality of events that may be interpreted as fantasy
come true. The latter leads to an obliteration of the
fantasy/reality boundary. This becomes especially a
problem in regard to the sensitizing fantasies that

create distortions through preconception in adult life. "Fantasy come true" experiences result in an undermining of the influence of reality. The idea that fantasy can control events encourages a shift of emphasis to primary process in fantasy oriented thinking and the use of evocative symbols. The child is left with the impression that if fantasies can come true, there is no telling what can happen. "If wishes were horses, beggars would ride", ceases to be an admonition in favor of restraint. Instead wishes and fantasies are trusted to be the source of things to be feared and of programs for progress that call vast energies to the pursuit of hollow crowns and of castles set in clouds that ignore the wind.

COMMUNICATIVE SYMBOLS AND MASTERY THROUGH FANTASY

Mastery through fantasy in play permits discharge and mastery of stress. Stress can be the result of unresolved conflicts. Stress can be the product of immediate pressures. The more that a child can be encouraged to use communicative symbols in the development of fantasy, play or dream, the more effective is the mastery of stress. Therefore the encouragement of communicative symbols is therapeutic. They help to achieve resolution of sensitizing fantasies through communicative mastery. Communicative symbols bring problems into an arena of consciousness shared by therapist and child. Evocative symbols are narcissistic. They leave the therapist to guess. Where there is a misunderstanding or a fantasy distortion or a sense of deprivation or a misinterpretation because of drive dominated wishes, communication with the analyst which uses mutually misunderstood evocative symbols establishes a zone of interaction in which realistic understanding is impossible. Shared communicative symbols make possible resolution of the situation to which the child is sensitive through insight. In the case of "Roy, the Boy Who would Be King", see bellow) discharge in play was effective in lessening his aberrant behavior. Only when he was able to communicate through the symbol "king" could his motivations be placed in consciousness and challenged and diminished. Only insight could diminish the slant of his beliefs to bring them into line with reality. Freud (1909) in noting the "psychological differences between the conscious and the unconscious" (p176) saw that "everything conscious was subject to a process of wearing-away, while what was unconscious was relatively unchangeable..." (P176). In order for what is unconscious to become conscious, contexts of reality must be followed as guides.

Fantasy formation during latency derives its contents from many sources. Recent events, comic book characters, culture heroes and the villains of history all take their places - in the helter-skelter palimpsest that is human memory. Upon, above, around, and below the emotional complexes of early childhood create subliminal impressions that beguile the ears and eyes of the therapist. This distorts the message. Similarities between memory elements cause fusions in recall that establish symbol like forms that lead the therapist astray.

They are subject to all the failings that befall
the communication of things past and remembered.
Such complexities add difficulty to child therapy.
The cognitive organization of memory in the child
is so different from that of the literate adult that
special listening skills must be developed. The
child in fantasy play is harder to understand than
the adult who remembers. Fantasy play and dreaming
are memory modalities that share qualities with free
association. However because of the primitive nature
of thought process in the child the associations
are looser. There is more primary process involved
(see below). The wandering mind of the child may
easily set the therapist to wandering as well.
This is especially disconcerting when one's free
floating attention, an informative study of one's
own reactions to the associations of the patient,
drifts unguided in the presence of the excessively
disconnected symbolic elements in the fantasies of
the child. Free floating attention becomes less of a
source of information. Instead it becomes a target
for attention that takes the therapist on an inner
directed track away from the manifest child. In the
meantime the child too drifts. His mind follows
source elements other than the progenitors of his
problems. The therapist in the absence of focus is
induced to drift also and to fall into "lulling".
(see Sarnoff 1976 Pages 243-6). When the child
finally comes to a word or situation that could be
interpreted, the therapist, his mind elsewhere, is
not ready to make the intervention. The therapist
must train himself to attend to the child's mental
content in the same way that a baseball outfielder
must not let up for a moment, though a ball may

come his way only once an hour. A poor defense taken against lulling is active participation by the therapist in the child's play on the level of the child. This contaminates content. A useful approach to lulling is the continuous diagnosis of fantasy content, psychosexual regressions and cognitive changes during the child's play. A search for the stimuli that give rise to such changes initiates forays into free floating attention ever refreshed by the input of the child's productions.

Fantasy Matures

Fantasy formation is the core of the process that produces play, manifest fantasy, and dreams. The structures of all three products undergo developmental changes. The predominant theme in this process is the movement of sources of manifest symbolic forms from the fantastic to the real. This is a part of the late - latency early adolescent maturational process that draws the attention of consciousness away from the fantasy of the subject towards the reality of the object. The child rises to adulthood on wings of reality. There are both normal and pathological aspects to the cognitive growth process. The degree to which reality testing replaces the sense of reality defines the success of the maturation and development of reality testing. The therapeutic approach to abnormal behavior must take into account both the content of fantasy and cognitive aberrations of symbolic form that force a breach in reality judgments. For instance, a child who acts out his fantasies in disruptive behavior because of a poor degree of displacement in symbol formation, and who cannot use fantasy to achieve comfort or delay, becomes a behavior problem. On the other hand, a child, gifted in fantasy play, with a similar latent fantasy is seen as creative.

JDS

Does the extended period of time each day that is devoted to video games by my patients take time and attention from working through in play and fantasy of stressful memories? Does extended button pushing distract from mastery of affect laden fantasies?

CAS

There is no question in my mind that children need alone time for creative play for working through of stress. Uninterrupted fantasy play using ludic symbols is an important factor in the potential therapeutic gain offered by childhood dynamic psychotherapy. Play under any circumstance can offer therapeutic gain.

Video games usually take time from creative play. There are exceptions to this rule. The story lines of video games can be used by the child to discharge violent tensions. Winning, recorded on the screen for all to see, can serve to reverse a latency age child's sense of inferiority in facing the adult world. Activities such as school achievement, sports, and toy construction can serve as well, with the addition of sharing positive achievements with others. The possibility of failure, which characterizes these contacts with outer things and beings, is greater than the positive outcomes inherent in the self steered goals and outcomes of childhood fantasy.

Child therapy sessions are primarily devoted to the resolution of unconscious conflict and affect laden memories. This does not rule out a secondary goal; the improvement of skills. Activities leading to enhanced skill and self esteem are important for children with low self esteem. Appropriately encouraged speed in accurate tapping on the remote control of a video game serves this purpose. Skill improvement gives more than pride. Applying the skill in new venues, such as typing and playing musical instruments, adds to personality potential.

RESOLUTION OF LATENCY AGE FANTASY

The conflicts of the prelatency and the latency years, whose distorting and sensitizing fantasies bring emotional discord to adolescent and adult life, are usually defused during the latency years. They are resolved through discharge and mastery through fantasy play or parental confrontation and education. This is a natural process. Should this process fail, distortions based on fantasy deflect a child's attention from conflict resolving realities, leaving the persistent influence of neurosogenic factors. Latency is a time when a reshaping of the self becomes possible. If as is said, "As the twig is bent so grows the tree.", then latency can be seen as a time for unbending. Bending factors carried by persistent distortions in fantasy can be diminished through dynamic child therapy. The normal resolution of conflict is adapted to this purpose, when the child is encouraged to free associate through fantasy play in sessions. This is achieved through enabling the child to abreact through playing out symbol based fantasy.

JDS

Can you tell us about other types of psychotherapy with children? How do they differ from dynamic psychotherapy.

CAS

There are many approaches to the troubled child. There are many therapeutically effective results claimed for them.

Such as-

Bribery- A frequently seen approach is bribery. Examples would be the eighteenth century approach of Goethe's mother, (see appendix one) who offered peaches in the morning to her children as a bribe to get them to stop having night fears. More recently a supervisee, who had recently arrived from Warsaw brushed aside my teaching with the announcement, "I promised him two quarters if he will behave himself."

Pastoral Guidance- Therapy underpinned by Platonic Dualism has a wide potential audience. Adding the power of God to attempts to bring behavior into line with cultural expectations enhances the therapist's expectation of reaching specific outcomes quickly. For instance dream interpretation is expanded in pastoral guidance to include such confrontations as "God is telling you in the dream how to better your life." Savary (1984) taught that dream interpretation is a way of "… consciously getting in touch with God's will and cooperating with it." (page 5)

Analytic psychology works with defenses and reminiscences as does dynamic therapy. In addition it postulates a flow into memory from a universal knowledge base that exists independently of the minds of living men, which shapes life choices and adjustment. Intrusions from this knowledge into dreams is recognized, valued, and used in interventions. The dynamic psychotherapist views this knowledge as information acquired from caretakers during the physio-verbal phase of knowledge encoding. Conscious recall of this data is accompanied by an affect of intense unchallengeable reality. Dynamic therapy with children is best done without challenges to these beliefs, for they are part of the mortar that shapes and holds together the family. Confrontation can precipitate unnecessary early termination. They represent reality to the family.

Therapeutically Effective Aspects Of Dynamic Psychotherapy with Children

"Dynamic" is a key word that will help me to clarify the boundaries of dynamic psychotherapy's territory from other types of psychotherapy. Dynamic therapy takes into account driven unconscious forces that are confronted and contained by defenses. Symptoms and behavior produced by this interaction are beyond the control of the child and interfere with a realistic adjustment. Analysis and resolution of distracting conflicts are the goals of dynamic therapy.

Many things that are therapeutic go on in the average playroom. Pedagogy gives knowledge. Water play enhances control. Building from kits improves self image. Games distract for the moment. Symbol drenched tales, repeatedly told in play, can lull the passively listening therapist. Songs offer experiences locked to expression by form.

Of all the activities that take place during dynamic child psychotherapy there are three that are the most productive. They keep the therapist alert. They offer him a way to use detected trends as gentle guides that save free association from the effects of the easy distractibility of childhood.

They are-

Gearing Interventions to the level of memory encoding that is in current use by the child.

Ludic Symbol Manipulation, that enhances free association; leading to play fantasies in which abreaction, catharsis, and reparative mastery of disruptive memories can be achieved.

Dream Interpretation through the adaptation of drawn or modeled dream elements for use as puppets, whose adventures expand and elaborate dreams into waking cathartic reveries.

Gearing interventions can aid communication.

Ludic symbol manipulation and dream interpretation open the gateway to knowledge of aberrant mental content, encourage free association, and encourage abreaction and mastery through play and interpretation by the therapist.

Ludic Symbol Manipulation

The ludic symbol is not a thing that inserts unique characteristics into new experiences. The ludic symbol itself is a passive entity that changes form and meaning to meet inner needs for wish fulfillment altered by the demand for compromise that is demanded by world and conscience. During the latency years, a found object can serve as a needed quasi-living thing, a ludic symbol, when reality has closed the door to satisfaction. During the latency years, the ludic symbol serves as an outlet, in loco persona when there are no real people available. Through suggestion, questions, offering toys or molded clay figures or turning drawn dream elements into puppets, the therapist can influence the choice of ludic symbol and create an interpretation that influences free association in play in a direction that enables abreaction and catharsis.

With the passing of the latency developmental phase the ludic symbol does not die. It changes to contribute, as did Proteus and Loki, a needed form. This occurs with every stage of encoding. For example the intermediate (transitional) object offers needed comfort to the lonely child during physiological encoding. Pictures remind. Badges reinforce ties to colleges. Compensatory fantasy in adult years make up for lost loves and failed ambitions. Older minds seek recourse in the hope that somewhere they will find a someone with whom they can waltz without tripping. Ludic symbols are given needed face and forms, much in the way that found objects are shaped by artists when creating art.

Adult minds, with sublimatory talent, can populate stories with ludic symbols, and can displace a troubling fantasy far from themselves onto the pages of a book or a sheet of music. They can free themselves of burdens by loading them into the minds of others. Such an escape into literature is not available to a child. Escape by reliving through a successful retelling of a painful experience of vulnerability in a fantasy is the childhood equivalent of adult sublimation.

Through history in myths, the vulnerability of a child, which dominates a child's awareness, is expressed in the many tales of "murder of the innocents", and the stories of Iphigenia, Joseph, and Hippolytus, which emphasize childhood seduction. Who could be more vulnerable than Hercules as a child when the serpent approached him? In mythic telling the child was given strength to kill the serpent. Note that in the retelling of frightening danger from the serpent, the mythmakers reversed the holder of the power. In many other tales of Hercules this theme is repeated. His labors are filled with dangers overcome. In the play "Alceste" he even wrestles death and wins.

THE DRAWINGS OF CHILDREN

The drawings of children can be used by a child therapist in a number of ways.

These are-

1. To estimate the intelligence of a patient.

2. To judge the level of development of a patient.

3. To pick up associational clues that can help the therapist give a therapeutic focus to a session.

4. To illustrate a dream or fantasy.

5. To serve as a flat physical representation of a dream, oneiric symbol content, which if cut-out and mounted as a puppet provide a toy image to be used in play to expand dream or fantasy content, through play and performance. This is a form of free association. Essentially this is a means of converting an oneiric symbol into a ludic symbol.

6. To introduce the possibility of organic factors to a differential diagnosis

Many illustrated books have been published over the last half century that deal with children's drawing. The ones that I have found to be most useful have been-

For Using Drawings To Determine Development, Age, and Maturity. Children transition from scribble-scrabble

to circles with legs at three and three quarters.. Memory encoding and word use follow a similar pattern. This parallel maturation of word and picture use, as a means of communication, may well be a manifestation of the cognitive march from the domination of narcissism in infancy to reality as a guide in adult life.

Di Leo, J.H. (1970) *"Young Children and Their Drawings"*, Bruner/ Mazel, NY

Fein, S., (1976) *"Heidi's Horse"*, Exelrod Press, Pleasant Hill, Ca.

Schildkrout, M.S., Shenker, I.R., Sonnenblick, M., (1972) *Human Figure Drawings in Adolescence"*, Bruner/ Mazel NY - Butterworth London.

For Using Drawings As Diagnostic Aids

Di Leo, J.H. (1973) *"Children's Drawings As Diagnostic Aids"* Bruner/Mazel, NY

Kaufman, B., Wohl, A., (1992) "Casualties of Childhood" Bruner/ Mazel NY

Wohl, A., Kaufman, Bobbie (1985) "Silent Screams and Hidden Cries" Bruner/ Mazel NY

Signs of pathology can be detected in figure drawings. For instance a child with a tear drawn below his eye evokes the thought that he is depressed. A drawing of a person with skin that is transparent so that the inner organs show is the drawing of a psychotic person. A drawing of a very small child relegated to a bottom corner of the page is depressed. A disjointed figure is a sign of organic pathology or great anxiety. A drawing of an enlarged body part indicates disease in that area.

Beware! What if the child with the tear knows someone with a dark nevus below his eye? What if the boy, who drew the transparent skin, is the son of a medical artist, whom the child idealizes and emulates? Drawings are like EEGs and child observation. In them diseases can be revealed by a sign that represents a disease. Such signs should be followed up with questions that will confirm or rule out the presumed diagnosis. When I was studying at the Hampstead Clinic in London, Anna Freud advised me that child observation tells little unless one knows what the child is thinking.

A reliable observation is that the presence of a neck in a figure is a sign of having achieved "latency". Another is the ten year old child's aptitude for producing figures, each of whose parts reflect the most common way of remembering the body part. The foot, hip, and face are drawn as seen from the side. The eye and the thorax are seen from the front. (See Di Leo 1970, pp 145-155)

Interpretive Use of Drawings with Interacting Protagonists

Fantasies or dreams, which are illustrated by a drawing or a three dimensional diorama using toys or clay figures can be adapted therapeutically. In asking a child to draw a picture, large pieces of paper are best. Space encourages more story and more characters. A picture that fills and exceeds the space and exceeds the borders of the paper is a sign of schizophrenia. In very young children a body part left out is not necessarily neglected. It can be that it was left out. The more details in a child's drawing, the more intelligent is the child. Eyes without pupils, think of poor relatedness.

Family drawing books offer diagnostic clues, through use of interpretation of what a child's drawing and its symbols could mean; for use in a therapy.

Burns, R.C. and Kaufman, S.H. (1970) *"Kinetic Family Drawings"*,

Burns, R.C. and Kaufman, S.H. (1972) *"Actions, Styles and Symbols in Kinetic Family Drawings"*, Bruner/ Mazel, NY

GUIDE TO FIGURE DRAWINGS

Figure 1 - Edna was a prepubertal girl, She had a younger brother. She had a dream in which she had been subjected to a procedure involving a ray source which was directed at her genitals.

Figure 2 - Illustrates the dream change in Edna's genitals produced by the ray in the dream. Her association to the picture that she drew based on the dream illustrates the effectiveness of drawing a dream in inducing further free associations to a dream. Note that passage of time with associated development can be carried over from a dream to a drawing.

Figure 3 - Illustrates the difference between prelatency figure drawing necks (absent) and latency age figure drawing necks (present).

Figure 4 - This is the drawing of a late latency boy. It illustrates what can be learned, gleaned, or guessed from a figure drawing. Follow up examination should seek confirmation of intuitive observations. -

He has a neck	= He is in latency.
There is no sexual differentiation.	= Not prepubertal
Eyes have pupils that are looking down and to the right	= impaired object ties.
There is a downward flow indicated by lines.	= He is sad. He is crying.
There is a dark mark on the left cheek.	= Could be a teardrop or a mark. Get his associations.
There are more details than is usual	= A sign of high intelligence.

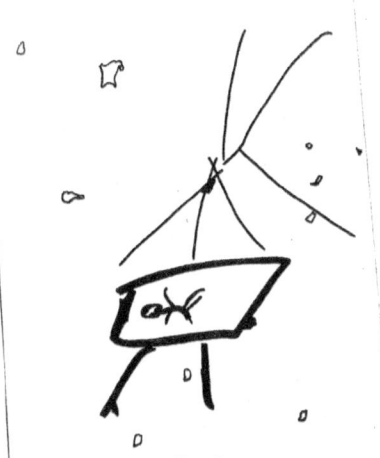

Figure 1

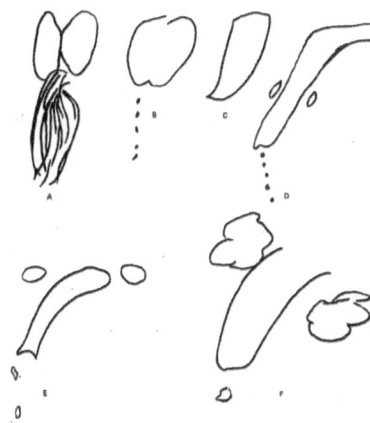

Figure 2

The dream had a definite effect on the analysis. She was able to speak more freely of her penis envy and to see its relationship to her depression and the overt anger she showed toward her brother. There is here a striking example of the unconscious meaning of the impending menarche. It reawakens bisexual fantasies. As such, as we will see, it stirs up aggression and confusion in the child.

Here is my vagina with a normal crack and peeing siss [Figure 2A]. Here it is bleeding. There is no more crack [2B]. Then it gets thinner [2C]. Then two pieces come out and make it look bent [2D]. Then the pieces move up and make the faucet controls [2E]. You know something, it looks like a penis [2F].

3

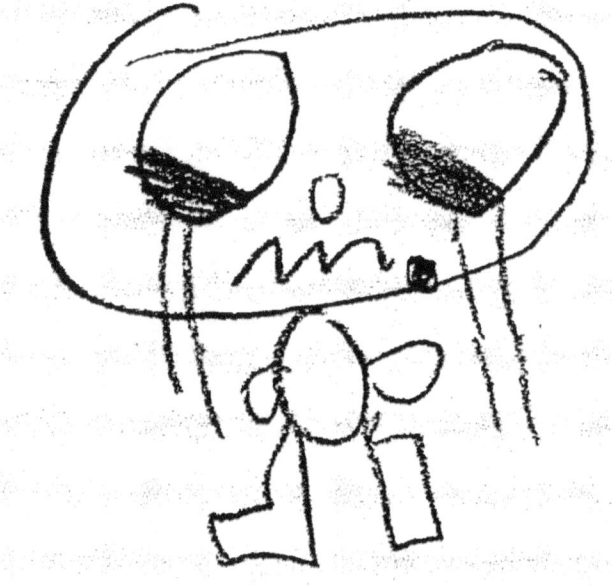

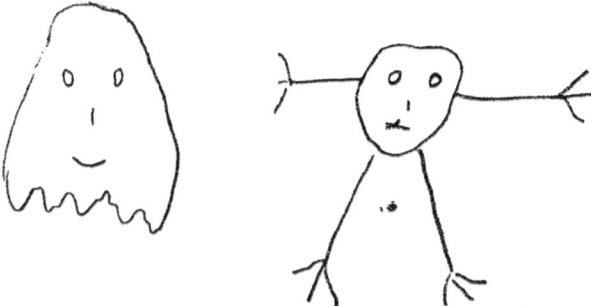

Figures without necks (4 and 5 year olds)

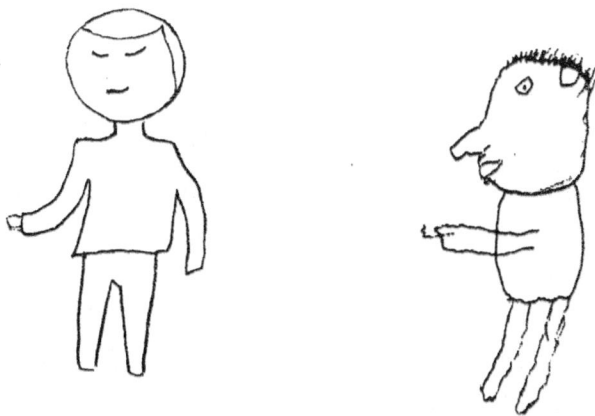

Figures with necks (8 year olds)   Figure 4

ASYMBOLIA

There are many forms of symbols. The simplest ones are single units, which represent directly more complex contexts of information. Their unimpaired meaning is known and shared by all who are initiated. They convey concepts. Words, signs, and signals can be used as simple symbols.

More complex symbols are representations, whose, relationship to meaning is hidden. Their numbers are legion. They are, in all but one example, consciously chosen. Examples are the symbols of secret codes, the symbols of religious mystery and the magic symbols of necromancers. The one type of complex symbols that stands apart from all the others are the Psychoanalytic symbols (oeneric, ludic, secondary, poetic, hypnogogic). Their unique characteristic is the ability to hide the meaning of their referents through serving as a countercathexis. Essentially this means that it diverts attention from its hidden meaning to the extent that it appears to stand alone. The hidden meaning is said to be repressed.

Examples are-

Oeniric (stage two REM state dream symbols). These manifest symbolic forms represent haptically encoded affect laden latent memory content, which has been displaced during sleep into a countercathectic entity. The latter draws attention away from latent content (repression); muting affect and preserving sleep. There is no conscious control over the choice of the oeniric symbol. There are two sources for REM state symbols. Those derived from haptic memory, and symbolicforms inspired by day residues, while they are still encoded in telereceptor memory.

Poetic representational symbols- The manifest forms are selected, after age twelve, from remembered experiences of the poet, (Example "Be prodigal, the lamp that burns by night, uses up its oil to give the world its light" is a call to sexual congress. (Shakespeare "Venus and Adonis.),

Ludic symbols (Piaget 1945) - (Ludens is the Latin word for play). - These symbols are actively selected by a child from external sources for use as conscious representations in fantasy play. Once selected, they are put to a test to see if they can be accommodated for use for surface expression of a secret meaning, or must be rejected as unsuitable. If accepted they become the content of childhood play, as occurs in play therapy. This characteristic can serve the therapist. It can serve as a portal for introducing guiding interpretations, based on insights gained from observing the ongoing content of a child's play. Through their introduction as toys, ludic symbols can serve, in the presence of low hormonal drive impetus, *in loco personas.* Abreaction through fantasy and cathartic discharge can be achieved through play containing ludic symbols. Adult writers of plays and novels can create using ludic symbols. Persistence of this skill is a unique talent.

For children the use of ludic symbols is time and development limited. For the child of two and a half years to four years of age the meaning of the ludic symbol is transparent. Then the therapist can obtain the hidden meaning merely by asking, and using the information obtained to counsel the parents. After the appearance of repression at four years of age, ludic symbols can be used for catharsis and abreaction through play in therapy. At eight years of age, with the introduction of abstract thinking, newly acquired representations gain influence. They are more and more people and less and less toys. Reality based representations place a limitation on fantasy input in daydreams and future planning. The child's thinking becomes assimilated to these representations of reality. The selection of ludic symbols from elements in reality becomes a portal for the introduction of reality considerations into the adolescent's thinking. Ludic symbols prepare the child for the reality dominance that influences object seeking with the increases in hormonal pressures that come with adolescence. With adolescence real personas come into range for the expression of unconscious fantasy needs. The usefulness of ludic symbols for children dwindles. Piaget (1945) notes that "about twelve the last forms of symbolic play come to an end." (p 287) Worth no more now than a tinker's dam, the ludic symbol falls from use. This is "Ludic Demise."

IMPAIRED SYMBOL USAGE

Psychoanalytic symbols sprout from mental states that are rich in anxiety, affect, and potentials for action that need be hidden from conscious attention. In the absence of symbols, or in the case of impaired symbolic usage, overt actions and felt affects dominate awareness. Where psychoanalytic symbols exist, one can find underlying secret wishes and blunted affects. Symbols can be used as markers that tell us that in the near unconscious, conflicts may be found. When the effectiveness of symbol usage is impaired, affects and impulses move toward awareness and action. There are only four references in the psychiatric literature to impaired symbolic usage (Winnicott (1953), Yaholem (1967), Libbey (1995), Sarnoff (2002). Among patients who have impaired symbol usage are chronic alcoholics, who deal with anxiety chemically, and the third type of ADHD (see Josie below), which should be looked for in latency age children, who do not produce states of latency.

Medications, which slow activity, growth and weight gain can counter the third type of ADHD. A psychotherapeutic technique is also available. It increases and enhances the use of ludic symbols in the ab-reactive fantasies of the latency state child. It enables the child to create ludic symbols to use in the creation of fantasies for use in the abreaction and resolution of the conflicts of the latency years An example of this technique is presented below.(see Josie.)

This psychotherapeutic technique offers to the child a personality based preparation for adjusting to expected future shifts in object seeking that occur in adolescence. The acquisition of adaptational personality defenses prepare the child for loss of ludic symbols as real drive targets increase during ludic demise. They enhance the introduction of real people to serve as drive objects. The hormone driven teenager is prepared, by test trials involving latency state ludic symbol laden fantasy during the latency years, for the reality stresses of adolescence.

Clinically Poor Symbolizing Function

Poor or absent symbolization predisposes a person to aberrant reactions. These include drive manifestations such as self directed anger when troubling ideation cannot be muted by displacement of attention to fantasy, dreams, and corrective future planning. People with poor symbolizing function tend to live out cycles. These consist of hope followed by disappointments, the impact of which lessens in time to permit the person to return with hope again and again to the same vulnerable situation. The interposition of mastery through dreaming, evocative fantasy, or the orderly creation of a new life through future planning involving realistic symbols can be insufficiently strong to produce options for change. The primary presenting symptom of a person with a symbol impaired character is recurrent depression that follows upon seemingly repetitive episodes of fate.

Pathological impairment of the symbolizing function occurs with brain damage, failure in development and psychological regressions. In the case of brain damage, for instance in the Kluver-Busey (1937) syndrome, the absence of the amygdala results in a lack of the interposed affect required to trigger cryptic symbol formation. Direct sexual, hunger, and aggressive drive expression result. In the aphasias Werner (1940) described regressed symbolizing function. He noted that there are "... certain psychopathological conditions in which the symbolic function has regressed..." (P 252) "... patients have not forgotten words as such, but they are quite unable to use them as displaced symbols.. They possess only a "dictionary meaning". With this type of aphasia, it is the intellectual ability to symbolize not the use of words for naming that is effected. The representation tends toward becoming a part of a "concrete natural situation" (p 253). The use of an isolated symbolism is beyond the powers of such aphasics. They may be capable of knocking at a door before entering the room, but be unable, as a pure fiction, to demonstrate the act of knocking. Luria (1968) has described mnemonists whose rich memories for concrete detail is accompanied by poor use of cryptic symbols.

There are impairments of the symbolizing function seen in feral children, stutterers, and deaf children, who experience a lack of example in their relative isolation,

In these people, interferences with the development of abstract thinking impairs the effectiveness of

any future symbolizing function. The impairment
is related to the difficulty caretakers have in
applying patience to teaching adult communication
skills involving time consuming repetition.

There are also youngsters with poor verbal memory
recall, in whom when the ability to establish
symbolic linkages through intrinsic characteristics
of referents and representations is lost.

The symbolizing function may be poorly developed or
subject to regression. Impairment of capacity for
delay, displacement, abstraction, symbolization, or
fantasy formation accompany this syndrome. Impaired
symbolizing function results in a person of unstable
character with an inability to generate patterns
of behavior consistently and constructively. In
these circumstances therapies require, in addition
to interpretation of unconscious content, specific
techniques aimed at strengthening the symbolizing
function and intercepting the factors that produce
the regressions, which destabilize reality oriented
cognitive organizations.

Yahalom (1967) reported a case of a woman with
poorly developed symbolic function. Her "...words
had not acquired the true symbolic function..."
resulting in "...many barriers to communication."
(p 377) She had "... critical confusions in sense
perception..." which "prevented her from forming and
using symbols..." (p 377). Such patients often do not
remember dreams. They give priority to evocative
symbols over communicative ones.

In reference to his patient Yahalom (1967) noted that "Symbols emerge through a process that transforms the characteristics of true images into representational percepts, and this transformation cannot take place unless one is able to "negate" the original object. Severely disturbed persons cannot do this" (P378) To form a symbol one must "detach (oneself) from all elements of emotional association with..." a memory. "Only then can (one) re-perceive..." the referent "...in the light of other less emotionally tinged memories and associations." (p 379) This is a description of the process of repression, when involved in psychoanalytic symbol formation.

Libbey (1995) described a non-symbolizing patient. "In these patients... symbol and symbolized are one." (p 82) As in Yaholom's case, there was no ability to "negate" the referent in favor of the representation and therefore impairment in the generation of symbols. She could not use dreams symbols in her analysis. The non-symbolizing patient does not recognize that the transference is a symbol of memories. As a result, the non-symbolizing patient is not open to "...the multiple possibilities for understanding the deep and complex meanings of personal experience." (p 72) including the transference. She recommends that in the treatment, emphasis be placed on discussions of the patient's "primal transference and the analyst's emotional position" (p 72). The process involves lending of the analyst's ego in creating symbols to represent the needs and referents of the patient that have been represented in a non-symbolized transference.

Early maturational fixation is implied by these authors as the origin of non-symbolization. The treatment of a child with this maturational fixation is presented elsewhere in this chapter (see below Josie). Psychotic paranoid transferences, in which the patient does not recognize his contribution to his own transference interpretation of the analyst's words or behavior, can result from a regression in the symbolizing function. The latter condition is characterized by irregular impairment of ability to separate representation from represented.

The Persistent Transitional Object

One process of impairment of maturation of the symbolizing function was described by Winnicott (1953). He introduced the concept that a child can cathect as a parent an object that stands for a missing parent. Such "...transitional phenomena are healthy and universal." (p 379) They are a means of dealing with separation in the infant. Ordinarily transitional objects such as teddy bears are given up when libidinal energies can be directed to non-parent caretakers. However a transitional object can persist into the latency years and adulthood as a non-symbol, which is not differentiated in the psychic reality of the child from the object it represents. In severely disturbed children the transitional stage does not give way to a fully effective symbolic thought process. The transitional stage persists and becomes anchored in an object (i.e. a fetish) "that serves as an image but not a symbol". (380)

The Hallucinated Concrete Object

Yahalom (1967) noted that the disturbed child is continuously driven to search for a concrete image, which offers a false sense of security. Without this safety he feels that all experiencing is unsafe; and he desperately settles for a fetish, a perversion, (the senseless repetition of a series of unworkable images) or a transference activated transitional object. All are manifestations of a desperate drive toward a hallucinatory concrete object (p. 380) with no differentiation of referent from representation and therefore are not a symbol. A functioning healthy observing ego can recognize that symbolic objects are representational and that substitute objects are not. Yahalom's patient's ego, being in a psychotic state, was not sufficiently developed to make this distinction.... she used this fictitious memory and the emotions, which she attached to it, to protect her from emotions, which she felt she should not endure. She knew of no other way to stave off inner catastrophe. (p. 380)

Josie –the Child with Impaired Utilization of Symbols and Failure to enter latency

At times a child has an absence of the ability to symbolize defensively. This interferes with fantasy play. Such children tend to have latency calm interspersed with episodes of marked anxiety, as opposed to excited behavior. Usually it is active symbolization that is missing. The child can passively use the symbols of others in the form of stories and TV dramas, for hours on end. She cannot, however, produce symbols on her own. Typically, such children fall into silence when they come upon material that is difficult to verbalize. This is in contradistinction to the shift into fantasy play that one normally sees in latency-age children. It is therapeutically useful to help these children to create unique personal symbols, so that they can develop fantasy play for use in therapy and life for the mastery of conflicts, humiliations, and fixations. How is this done? One technique is to introduce clay figures, doll figures or drawings to represent the situation being described by the child at the moment he became silent. The next step is to ask the child what happens next, or even to suggest what may happen, using doll figures to illustrate the suggestion. As with most work, which deals with cognitive growth in children, the symbolic potential of these children exceeds their functional capacity. This can be harnessed for therapeutic gain.

Therapy of a Child with Poor Symbol Formation

Josie was a seven year old second grade student. She had shown anxiety during back-to-school activities at the end of the previous summer. She had had a similar experience the prior year with rapid resolution of anxiety. Her behavior during preparation for school included awakening her parents at four AM on a Saturday to go over the preparations for dressing for Monday morning. Six weeks into the school year, the problem became so severe that her parents brought her for therapy.

In therapy sessions, she reported in the minutest detail, the events of the school day. She did this with her parents too. If they could not listen, she became overwhelmed with anxiety and a sense of urgency. The parents could not recall a single spontaneous fantasy of the child. Josie had always been a nagging child. She could not occupy herself when there was no structure. There was a continuous need for attention from the parents.

She reported to me that she had to tell her parents what happens in school, because the voice of a lady told her to. She didn't know who the voice was. She was clearly without access to spontaneous play. She presented no fantasies. In therapy sessions she waited silently for me to speak. She said nothing spontaneously. She drew no pictures spontaneously. She was well oriented. There were no evidences of general cognitive impairment. There was an obvious maturational lag manifested in the absence of superficial evidences of a repression-oriented symbolizing function used in the service of latency fantasy discharge. She could remember no dreams save those, which repeated recent traumatic experiences or frightening television movies. She enjoyed watching television but could recall only exciting events, never full stories or story lines. Explosions, fights, and isolated episodes of magic on TV sitcoms were all that held her interest. She had a fear of robbers. She provoked the attack of peers. Her capacity to pay attention in school in support of learning was supported by adequate latency ego mechanisms of restraint.

Her teacher tended to yell at the pupils in her class. This recreated the home situation for Josie and stirred great anger in her. She feared to show it to the teacher, containing her anger until she returned to her home. She dealt with her acute distress by insisting upon parental attention to a reliving of the trauma of the school day. The amount of aggression leveled at the parents at these times was so great that she dealt with her motivation regressively, assigning the cause of her behavior to a voice rather than to herself. She was incapable of dismantling the memory of traumatic events and reorganizing and synthesizing them into highly symbolized and displaced stories. She therefore approached stresses bereft of skills, through which she could gain succor or revenge without threatening the situation in which she wished to continue to function well (school). She did not have available the structure of latency that could permit this.

The dynamics of her current state is best described as acute disorganization in an individual who was experiencing an ineffective latency as a result of inadequate symbol formation. Although some calm had been achieved in school, the absence of the structure of latency made it impossible for the child to remain calm in the face of ordinary stresses, where structure was minimal. If the child were to be helped at all, psychotherapy had to aim at creating a symbolizing function, which she could use as a safety valve to deal with stress. The root of her problem was that she had become an unimaginative child with no apparent psychoanalytic symbols.

In falling from consciousness, a traumatic event is stripped of its outer garments (words) and is hidden in the mind only as the idea of what it had meant to the person who experienced the event. There are no words in the part of memory of which I speak. There are only ideas of things. The part of the mind which contains such memories is called the *system unconscious.* It is a characteristic of this part of the memory that events which carry much meaning become linked to memories from the past, which are related i.e. the overwhelming yelling of the teacher and the yelling of the child's parents). The recent event and the past events in combination increase each other's momentum in seeking a conscious representation which will provide an opportunity for reliving, working through, and putting to rest the trauma. As such they are a source of discomfort. The more discomfort, the more does the complex of ideas of things acquire the quality that will attract consciousness.

The organ which opens the door to consciousness we call the *percept consciousness.* Eventually, the disquieting event and its comrades in arms knock at the door of consciousness and demand entrance. How can they be admitted? This is a land of protocol. Only thoughts that are dressed as words may enter here. Fortunately, there is an anteroom near the door to consciousness. We call it the *system preconscious.* Here there are garments in the shape of words and nonverbal visual symbols, which hide the private parts of the ideas of things, while cloaking them in styles and forms which are admissible into polite society. Once so attired, the concepts and ideas enter into the area of awareness which we call the *system consciousness.*

During the latency years, the use of symbols, fantasies, and masking is a primary adjustment technique in working through traumatic events. This was not so with Josie. A trauma remained with her, and she remained conscious of it. She could not deal with it through symbols and substitutes. These skills she had to acquire. Her way of dealing with trauma reflected a failure in development of psychoanalytic symbols as a means of reintroducing past trauma into consciousness in a form sufficiently masked to permit working it through and mastering it without overwhelming her with an affect that would have paralyzed the process.

Fortunately, she had some rudiments of psychoanalytic symbol formation. She could participate passively in the psychoanalytic symbols of others (passive symbolization). She could take over the stories of others to fill her nightmares. She was able to express her affects through the excitements of television programs. Still her capacity to form symbols was limited and she could not use them to achieve a competent latency age adjustment.

What could be done about this? An attempt had to be made to strengthen her repression and provide her with a capacity to form of displaced symbol oriented fantasies. In this way she would be enabled to acquire the calm resources of latency. Her ability for passive symbolization was used as a resource for the therapist, in developing her capacity for the development of psychoanalytic symbols.

The therapy began with a child who sat anxiously and silently throughout each session. When spoken to about her problems, she answered politely, but never spoke more than a few words. I began to ask her about home, friends, her sister, and school. She described her need to talk about school to her parents. I pursued this, encouraging her to talk to me about school. I noticed that there were times when she would cut short her answers to my questions. This occurred especially when I asked her about her feelings and thoughts about her teacher? "You stopped talking in the middle of a sentence; did your thoughts stop?" "No," she said, "I know them; I can't say them."

Here was a manifestation of anxiety in response to a specific event.

I stepped over to my doll house and obtained a toy table, two toy chairs, a girl doll, and an older man doll. I set them up on the table at which we sat in an arrangement which duplicated our own seating arrangement. In essence I had created symbols for her to adapt passively to her own preoccupations. She called the doll "Lisa". "Do you know anyone named Lisa?" I asked. "No," said Josie, "I made it up." She looked a bit shy and uncertain. An event had happened in the therapeutic situation to which a therapist should have been alerted by symbol theory. She had created a substitute masked form of an original referent. She had actively produced a masking symbol. I said to Josie, "Lisa, what happens in your school on a typical day?" Josie began to answer for Lisa, recounting her own experiences. When we arrived at the point where I asked her feelings when with the teacher, she fell into silence. But I was ready. She could live her fantasies passively through the stories of television characters. I would provide her with characters through whom she could tell her own story. I reached for the doll house and brought out seven child dolls and two adult women dolls, plus some doll furniture. Josie caught the idea of the play, and using the substitute objects, I had provided, played out the following story.

In a classroom, a child makes a simple request. (I am to speak for the child; she speaks for the teacher. I do not speak except when given specific words to say by Josie.) The teacher refuses the request. When the child complains, the teacher begins to yell. At first all the children are frightened. Then they all rise up, advance upon the teacher, and kill her.

In many guises, she repeated the same story in the months that followed. During this time, the parents noted an improvement in her behavior. The nagging stopped. The voice of the lady was heard no more. Tension occurred only on Sundays preceding school. One day in the playroom, she noticed a tiny sarcophagus containing a tiny mummy. It was made of dried clay. It was a remnant of a long-ago analysis of a child who made her own dolls to relate her fantasies. I told her this. She asked me to get some clay. I produced it from a nearby cabinet and handed it to her. She mushed it and rolled it and

squashed it and then put it aside to play the game
of the school situation.

In the next session, I began to mold the clay in
my hand. Josie's therapeutic gain had reached the
point that she could passively adapt dolls set in a
context by me to tell a story that was so close to
the original that the meaning was hardly masked.
This was only part of the way to real symbol
formation. To achieve that, she must produce her
own symbols. I held the shapeless piece of clay in
my hand so that she could see it clearly. Then I
asked, "What am I making? See how quickly you can
guess it." She peered at the clay and said, "a man."
So I made it into a man. The next piece of clay she
saw as a dinosaur. Dinosaur it became. Then she
tried her hand, producing another dinosaur. She had
made the jump from the use of ready-made symbols
to express fantasies to creating her own symbol.
Now could she use these for working through her
problems? The answer came quickly. OShe put a blue
piece of paper and some paper trees into a small
box and then arranged the figures in the box. "Write
down a story about it," said I. "Okay," said she, and
she did. (This case is presented more extensively in
Sarnoff (1976 P 185.) With the introduced capacity
for delay, latency states became possible.

DEFINITIONS OF EVOCATIVE AND COMMUNICATIVE SYMBOLS

Evocative Symbols

Intrinsic to the nature of evocative symbols is the selection of a symbolic signifier to represent unconscious referents without regard for the communicative or aesthetic value that it has for an audience. Often when a trauma or affect laden fantasy figure has been repressed, the affect remains free floating in the memory systems. Freud (1909) noted that in that circumstance "We are not used to feeling strong affects without their having any ideational content, and therefore, if the content is missing, we seize as a substitute some other content which is in some way or other suitable..."(p176) Highly personal and idiosyncratic symbolic forms selected in this way, hide the identity of the latent content. These symbolic signifiers evoke - for the benefit of the egocentric aspects of the individual - inner feelings and experiences. Evocative symbols represent a victory for narcissism. The product of this repetition is mastery through momentary personalized gratifying play. In each case already mastered fantasies and feelings are re-experienced at the expense of reality.

Communicative Symbols

Intrinsic to the communicative symbol is selection of representations based on the sense of reality, knowledge and needs of the audience. Communicative symbols represent a victory for reality, altruism, and non-egocentric influences. These symbolic signifiers work for the benefit of object relations. The transformation of fantasies by changing symbol content and symbolic forms to match the ways of the world enhances object relations. Through such fantasies, contact with the world of reality of the therapist can be achieved, interpretations made, and discussion initiated. Working through then becomes possible. Past traumas can be de-emphasized and reparatively mastered and processed. A psychotherapeutic strategy that encourages the development of mature symbols and symbolic fantasy play in therapy sessions is based on these theoretical considerations. By way of example, see the case of Roy ("The Boy who Would Be King"). A part of the shift from evocative to communicative symbols is the selection of the therapist as a ludic symbol equivalent. This is an intense form of transference. Although it may occur during latency, it is strongest during early adolescent removal, when one must be alert for sexual acting out of the transference.

When the march of symbols has reached the point that real figures can be recruited to populate fantasies, and the communicative pole dominates selection of symbols, and situations are constructed and interpreted on the basis of reality testing derived from operational thinking, the cognitive underpinnings of the ability to fall in love have been attained and the task of latency has been completed.

While working with early adolescents in therapy, the child's level of attainment in the use of communicative symbols should be evaluated. Psychotherapeutic strategies should be developed that will enhance these cognitive skills. (see Sarnoff (1987B) pp171 - 222)

BEHAVIORAL NEOTENY

The maturation and development of children are influenced by a multitude of factors, each of which must be considered in understanding emotional growth errors that produce behavioral variants and pathologies in childhood and adolescence. Poor example setting can alter adjustment and behavior. Strong affects can distract a child from the exercise of skills afforded by advancing cognition. Persistence in memory of early trauma and regression in the face of frustration can result in sustained immature behavior patterns. Innate potentials inherent in maturation are shaped by genetic forces. Juvenile cognition persisting into adulthood produces an immature adult who cannot gain from social phase specific educational opportunities. Darwin (1872) described such a "loss of the adult stage of development" in species, which reach reproductive potential "before they acquire their perfect characters" (p 113).

Budiansky (1991) has extended this concept to include behavioral characteristics and object relations. He points out that "... variation within a species is normally limited... by basic rules of genetics and development. But there is one source of enormous variation within a species..." "The range of variation in any adult population is miniscule compared with the differences that separate the average adult from the average juvenile.... If the genes that govern this development process change in such a way that adulthood is reached before the normal process of development is complete, youthful characteristics will be locked in. This process is called neoteny..." (p 20) "Neoteny" may be manifested by the presence of behavior, that is derived from genetically controlled persistence of immature cognitive structure and function into adulthood, such as concrete thinking, magical thinking, narcissistic object relations, primary process dominance, and dominance of the evocative pole in symbol formation. Budiansky (1991) illustrates this by referring to the persistence of dependency and ability for cross species object ties, which exist in the object relationships of infantile forms of animals, who become capable of domestication as adults.

The transient neurotic symptoms of childhood are products of the ever-changing cognition that accompany growth. Transformations of cognition are normally inherent in the maturation of personalities. Failure to transform introduces a potential to lock in immature forms of cognition and relatedness, to the detriment of adult life. When this is encouraged either by genetic limitations on progress or receptive parental or social attitudes, persistence occurs. In the human species this can produce large populations with maladaptive personality features to which a tolerant and humane society may chose to adjust. In individual personalities this contributes to the formation of fixed immature cognitive structures. The fixed nature of these structures contributes to the chronic nature of neurotic symptoms in the adult. In this regard it is of interest to recall Schilder's (1938) definition of "...symbolism as an experimentation which is retarded in comparison with the general state of development, in the perceptive and emotional sphere." P25

In addition to interpretation and working through of fantasy, it is beneficial in child therapies to encourage patterns of cognition (i.e. abstract memory systems, symbolic forms, and reality testing) that will enhance adaptive potential in adulthood.

UNIT FIVE-

LUDIC SYMBOLS

BIOLOGICAL SOLDIER DWARFS SEEK HAVEN FROM THEIR ISOLATION, IN FANTASY AND PLAY SYMBOLS THAT SERVE AS PARTNERS IN THE RESOLUTION OF PAST INDIGNITIES.

Use of Fantasy Symbols During Dynamic Psychotherapy with Children

LUDIC SYMBOLS

INTRODUCTION

During the latency years (six to twelve), fantasy, expressed in play, is the primary defensive response to the power of the adult populated world. Fantasy play, encouraged during childhood psychotherapy gives access to this response. The symbols of fantasy play are called ludic symbols [see Pages 90 and 173 of Piaget (1945)]. They take form from the toys and plastic objects of the well equipped playroom. They can be seen in the child's drawings that have been cut out and mounted to use as puppets. They are the clay figures that have been molded to fit the child's recognition.

Ludic symbols can be introduced, influenced and modified by a therapist. This is a form of interpretation that opens a gateway through free association to affect laden unconscious content. Once expressed in fantasy play troubling content can be reparatively mastered, or remain unresolved to reappear as repetition compulsion. The haptic oneiric symbols of dreams are not introduced by the therapist. Their source is in the haptic memory of the sleeping child. Through a therapeutic manipulation the oeniric symbol can be converted into a ludic symbol. As the child reports a dream, the therapist asks the child to draw the dream. The drawn dream figures are then cut out and mounted on board with a base. The child is then encouraged to expand on the dream using the figures produced. Associations follow.

Mastery of ludic fantasy can be achieved through erosion by abstract constructions, offered by the therapist that identify themes. This reduces a ludic symbol, an entity, which, had been related to as a living, close, feeling being, into a denizen of the cold and distant world of words.

Mastery of ludic fantasy can also be achieved by abreaction, which occurs while the therapist listens quietly. Play fantasy is in essence an effort by the child to relive tragic loss of face, experienced when he felt humiliated. The ludic fantasy of play is an attempt to relive such a negative past event with a child positive outcome. The past is less painful thereafter and less prone to shape feelings and behavior. Discharge of drive feelings is concurrently achieved through catharsis.

With adolescence, ludic symbols give way to real people, as objects in fantasy. Play gives way to verbalization. Symptoms give way to character based behavior. Ludic demise occurs. During ludic demise the therapist can offer confrontations, which shape the child's approach to reality behavior.

LUDIC SYMBOLS AND LATENCY STATES

Ludic symbols are the symbols that dominate
children's play during psychotherapy play sessions.
Ludic symbols can serve in place of reality objects
as protagonists with whom the child can process
remembered trauma and abreact affect laden fantasy.

All symbols consist of a representing word, feeling,
or image, and a represented entity in memory.
A symbol is created when the child recruits a
word (for instance) to serve a role in one of
his fantasies. He practices its effectiveness in
being a representation of any entity in memory.
The recruited word, if successful, is then used
to represent an element from a forbidden story, in
search of expression, cathartic discharge through
re-experiencing, and abreaction producing oblivion.
Thus is created a fantasy which contains a word
pair (secret and communicative) that both hides and
reveals painful unconscious content. The recruited
word in awareness is called a ludic symbol, if it can
serve to express and dissipate through corrective
reliving in fantasy the origins of affects linked
to the symbolic word pair. A ludic symbol is an
imitation of life. It can absorb and dissipate affect,

the way that real people as objects of aggression absorb rage. The memory encoded element of the word pair becomes less restless, and less impelling in seeking aware attention through displacement to expression through a symbol.

The affect linked unconscious (repressed) element becomes attenuated in its strength and lost to awareness. It lies quiet in the cellars of memory. Shorn of affect, it is forgotten. What is unique to the ludic symbol is its status as an imitation of life that is strong enough to serve as a surrogate for reality, a whipping boy, a Judas goat; essentially it is an object for expressing love or revenge in the service of reliving, through abreaction and cathartic discharge during play. Dream symbols can serve a similar function. However REM dream symbols can not be controlled. Ludic symbols can be controlled in the service of the patient's needs. In fact selection of the representation becomes, throughout the latency years, an early portal for interpretive intervention and informed input by a therapist. The child therapist can participate in the selection of symbols that will lead to unconscious content by asking about dream content, turning dream drawings into puppets to use in stories, and patient recognition based clay modeling to be placed into dioramas. A second portal opens at the age of eight, when abstracting capacities gain strength. Then, associations based on the intrinsic characteristics of things described, can be generated in response to a therapist's request that the child expand on a manifest reference.

Remembrance of repressed stresses and things past come to light.

Developmental Stages of Ludic Symbolism

Ludic symbols appear at all stages of life. They appear in the works of dreamers, poets, playwrights. They serve sublimation. They make the state of latency possible when it is needed.

THE LATENCY STAGES OF LUDIC SYMBOLISM

PRE- THROUGH EARLY LATENCY

TWENTY-SIX MONTHS TO EIGHT YEARS

LUDIC SYMBOLS during Pre- through early Latency are entities such as toys that are selected from the ambient world on the basis of concrete similarity of predicates. They can serve abreaction. They are selected for their ease of accommodation to self centered narcissistic orientations. Before they are used as ludic symbols their ability to accommodate their use to self needs was practiced. This portal from the ambient world to patient thought content in free association is available to a therapist interested in interpreting or advancing a trend or encouraging abreaction.

LUDIC SYMBOLS DURING LATE LATENCY

-EIGHT YEARS TO TWELVE YEARS -

During late latency the relationship between a ludic symbol and that which is represented is based on intrinsic similarities. The child's tendency to accommodate new experiences to his preconceptions is diminished. This is a result of the influence of abstract thinking in reinforcing assimilative pressure from the real world. At this portal, the therapist can introduce interpretations about similarities between fantasies and generally known tales, and point out trends of similarity that are coming to the fore in the play therapy. In essence, this encourages more focused free associations. Phobic entities that threaten take on a humanoid form (i.e. witches replace goblins.)

LUDIC DEMISE

-TWELVE YEARS TO FIFTEEN YEARS-

Increased hormonal pressure, social pressure, physical maturation and the presence of real objects at twelve years of age reinforce assimilation of private needs to public availability. Love relationships are shaped by movie imagery. Ludic symbols become less important than reality entities for solving problems of mood and memory. At fifteen years, teamwork and the needs of the object take priority. This further intensifies reality influenced assimilation.

LUDIC SYMBOLS IN LATE LATENCY
- EARLY ADOLESCENCE

The Unheralded Turning Point

Much attention is devoted to latency and adolescence. They are treated in theory as though they are distinct phases with finite beginnings and endings. During active therapy sessions this distinction does not hold up. (See Sarnoff October 1987). The therapist should be alert to pathology and aberrations that intrude on development during the transition phase between latency and adolescence.

Late latency-Early adolescence begins at eight years of age. "Reversal" (Piaget) of goal occurs at its beginning. Engaging the world, through narcissistically accommodating its reality to personal and previously learned needs, dwindles. With reversal, reality comes to call the tune. Reality and its needs are engaged and assimilated, becoming the primary guide for developing impressions, hopes, and future plans. Early adolescence ends at about fifteen years of age, when the needs of reality that dominate interpersonal relations focus on

capacity for teamwork and satisfaction of the needs
of potential love objects.

Within this seven year period of gradual transition,
there is one year, from twelve to thirteen years of
age that contains a sharp turning point. Clinically,
during this turning point year, one sees the
following signs-

PHYSICAL- growth spurts, increase in hormonal
secretion with primary and secondary sexual
characteristics and increased drive pressures, first
ejaculation (See Sarnoff 1976), menarche (see Sarnoff
and Hart 1971c) with increased verbalization, and
transition of the site of therapy from the playroom
to the talking room.

OBJECT SEEKING- Voyeurism (Peeping Thomism), crushes
as an early phase of falling in love, a shift from
cathexis of fantasied objects to a search for real
objects, reactive depression.

REGRESSION- Psychosomatic symptoms (anorexia nervosa
[see Sarnoff (1982)], colitis appear.

SUBLIMATION- abstract poetry colored by projection
appears. (See Sarnoff 1972b).

These changes in the working ego and its products
can be detected during therapy sessions. For example
the change of the site for therapy from the playroom
to the consulting room and the shift in activity
from play to verbalization is obvious. Physical
changes, which are associated with this transition,
are demanding realities. Keeping up with them is

a primary pressure of the period. The patient, now larger, is no longer required to be passive; he is no longer a biological soldier dwarf. Real objects match his size and strengths. With growth, fantasy is no longer mandatory. Real objects offer satisfactions. The need for ludic symbols dwindles. For those who can seize the day, the world is theirs. For those, who are sorely stressed, regression to the physiological level of encoding offers a haven from progress and its stresses.

For those whose sense of reality interprets and responds to stresses through misunderstanding, fulfillment lies beyond reach. Frustrations, humiliations, insults, and losses pass through gates to memory that close behind them. There is no way out for those whose ingrained negative self image has been reinforced by insult. Reality is distorted, comfort is rejected. Moments of stress and their affects remain unabated in memory. Suppression and displacement resulting in repression encapsulate them away from awareness at great expense of attention and energy. There is some relief, when displacement into symbols create new forms acceptable to awareness, and abreaction through metaphor dissipates their force. Humiliating episodes held in memory with little change in form or content are disturbing. They become the day residues of dreams. These restless affect laden memories rise, like bugs in bubbles rise through water; toward redress in fantasy. A successful reliving of humiliations in awareness, guided by fantasy, offers in its retelling a quieting resolution for pain.

For those with a good self image a positive outcome
for the relived moment is supported. Such an outcome
is called reparative mastery. For those whose self
image denies them recompense, the re-fantasied
reminiscence is useless except as a source of
pain. Such failure draws energies and time from
confrontations with reality. Hope becomes hopeless,
when linked to repetitions of fantasies that are
doomed to fail. Such an outcome, which can persist
through adulthood is called repetition compulsion.

**Gearing Therapeutic Interventions to the Current
Active Memory Encoding Phase That the Patient Is
Using**

*The following charts are offered as an aide for
identifying operative memory encoding phases.*

Chart one

PHYSIOLOGICAL MEMORY

(Somatic Protosymbols)

ENCODING	ENCODED In	EXPRESSED	REPRESSED Attention
Through Physical Changes	Potential Organic Responses	Manifest Physical Signs (i.e. Hives)	Displaced to the Symptom Suppresses Awareness

AGE: PRENATAL tO ADULTHOOD in RESPONSE tO STRONG STRESS.

IMPACT ON FUTURE: PTSD VULNERABILITY

SYMBOLS - NONE

Psychosomatic symptoms become more apparent during late latency - early adolescence. During that phase outlets through ludic fantasy become less important with the availability of real drive gratification objects. The transition to reality sources is stressful. A potential response to pubertal reality stress is regression to the use of violent verbal fantasy. This response can be suppressed by activation of somatic expression. If a concomitant loss of the potential for recognition of patient aggression that words carry is lost during a therapy session, an effective psychotherapeutic maneuver that returns the patient to verbal content and associations is the question, "What were you thinking just before the hive appeared?"

Chart two

AFFECT LINKED WORDS

ENCODING	ENCODED	EXPRESSED	REPRESSED
As words linked to Physio-logical affect	As a real basis for identity	Incontra-vertible	none,

AGE of Acquisition: TWENTY SIX MONTHS TO THREE YEARS

IMPACT ON FUTURE: Continues through states of fixation or regression. Under stress affect linked words are activated strongly. Their linked incontrovertible sense of reality strengthens personal identity, religious beliefs, and politics.

IMPACT ON THERAPY: Direct challenge or confrontation by the therapist has little effect. This phenomenon is important in understanding group psychology.

SYMBOLS: Concrete transparent representations.

Chart three

SHARED MEANINGS THROUGH SHARED WORDS

ENCODING	ENCODED	EXPRESSED	REPRESSED
As reality derived from shared interpretation with a mentor.	In panels used for recognition of new Experience.	Shared not conscious-ness of culurally recognized reality.	when to shared

AGE: BEGINS AT THREE YEARS

IMPACT ON FUTURE: Shared meaning equals conscious sharing.

SYMBOLS - transparent

Chart four

SHARED REALITY

AGE: Four Years

Impact on therapy: Shared references make understanding each other possible.

IMPACT ON FUTURE: Introduces the possibility of creating a shared reality based on repeatability, transmissibility and verifiability.

Impact on therapy: Good for relating. Poor for challenging occult symbolized ideas.

SYMBOLS - Repression aides in making symbols less transparent. Fantasies are used for Ludic resolution. Free association through play becomes the primary therapeutic

Modality in childhood psychotherapy.

Chart five

CONCRETE THINKING

ENCODING	ENCODED	EXPRESSED	REPRESSED
Associated	In surface	Felt to be	Concrete
With concepts	defined	real	thinking
that are super-	Mode of Barbara		
ficially similar	reality clusters		

Mode of Barbara: Indians are swift.
                 Antelopes are swift.
                 Therefore Antelopes are Indians

AGE: Six to Eight Years

Impact on therapy: Logical intervention is weak. Ludic play induced mastery of stressful memory takes priority.

IMPACT ON FUTURE: Fixation at this point prepares a child for a limited role in society.

SYMBOLS - Strong hiders of meaning. The link of the symbol to latent content is arbitrary and based on superficial similarities.

Chart six

ABSTRACT THINKING

ENCODING	ENCODED	EXPRESSED	REPRESSED
Associated	with	Felt to be	Counters
	related		
With concept	concept	real	repression
clusters	clusters		
that are insically similar			

The acquisition of Abstract Thinking begins at eight years of age with ability to understand proverbs reached at eleven years of age.

IMPACT ON THERAPY: Abstract verbal interpretations become possible. The use of abstract thinking by the therapist is a pedagogical technique that enhances the patient's growing skills through identification and introjection..

IMPACT ON FUTURE: Abstract thinking is necessary for surviving in modern society. There are primitive societies that forbid it.

SYMBOLS: Contribute to psychosis, phobia formation, and hysterical neuroses.

Creative sublimations are populated by cryptic symbols. These are necessary for adjustment and for understanding intellectual phenomena.

LUDIC SYMBOLS AND LUDIC SYMBOL EQUIVALENTS THROUGH THE STAGES OF LIFE

Ludic symbols serve a universal need. At every age there is a move toward surface awareness from repressed memory; of affect laden experiences involving unfulfilled expectations and lost loves. Painful affect draws awareness to these memories. The pain of the affect forces the memory toward displaced representation, which softens the rawness of the memory. The altered representation is the psychoanalytic symbol.

Each stage of life offers a form of substitute representation that is suitable for a person's age. Each substitute offers a possibility of comfort and resolution, and serves to serve a longing for release from the pain that had impelled the memory toward awareness. During the years of latency and early adolescence, fantasy expressed in play serves this form of outlet. The child is too small and inexperienced to reverse past discomforts. School achievement, sports, and oft told tales of adventure help, but carry the possibility of losing. Play symbols on the other hand, can be manipulated to provide expectations of unfailing success in reliving and correcting past losses.

The symbols of play fantasy are called ludic symbols. [Ludic is the Latin word for play.] The symbols of play fantasies are regarded as though they are real entities, which can react to the needs of the child. They are the toys in the playroom. They are the thoughts in latency age fantasy given form. Other stages of life also offer objects to serve in lessening longing.

.Stage One- For the "mewling and puking" infant there are physiological sensations whose recall turns encoded memory into comforting reality "for a little while". With the establishment of ego boundaries, blankets and dolls serve as ludic symbol equivalents. They represent portable substitutes for the not always available breast and parent.

Stage Two- For the "whining schoolboy" of the latency age period, who is mobile, but cut off by his size from redress in reality, there are fantasies and **play,** whose ludic symbols offer themselves as tools for play therapy content, such as revenge.

Stage Three- For the "lover" of late adolescence there are drives, size, and coy partners to serve and pursue. Success is not always guaranteed in reality for this call to action. Weakened ludic symbols wait in reserve like Frederick Barbarosa, sleeping in his cave until calls to action awaken him. When needed "woeful ballads made to his mistress' eyebrows", and stories to be shared, serve abreaction, catharsis and the resolution of remembered stress.

Stages Four and Five- For the adult "soldier' and the wiser adult "justice" gratifications and resolutions await in reality. For them, unresolved hopes and conflicts find catharsis and resolution of remembered stress in passively experienced stories, which have been written by people, who have retained skills in producing ludic symbols. When performed, these stories are rightly called **plays**.

Stage Six- For the person in retirement, "a world too wide for his shrunk shank" places reality beyond his grasp. Turning inward he relives the longings of the past through dwelling on ludic equivalents in the form of all the could-ovs, would-ovs, and should-ovs that he could call up from the past to fill empty moments, when the grand-children are gone.

Stage Seven- For the person who has entered "second childhood" and awaits "mere oblivion", the mind dwells on personal reflections on fears about the afterlife (eschatology).

In a unique reversal, ludic symbol equivalents offer comfort in the face of fears of the future after-life, in place of offering comfort in the bitter face of yesterday's memories.

I am indebted to William Shakespeare for the many phrases, above in quotes, from his **play** "As You Like It" (Act IV Scene 7) in which the distinct characteristics of the seven stages of man, were described.

THE STRENGTH OF LUDIC SYMBOLS
BRINGS OUT THE TRANSFERENCE

ROY, THE BOY WHO
WOULD BE KING

For the prelatency and latency age child, the use of verbal interpretation undoes the defenses that permit the calm, and educability of the state of latency to exist. Dreams and drawings, fantasy and therapeutic play serve to help the child revisit trauma and relive feelings. Through reliving in masked form, a hoped for diminishing of the repressed fantasy's ability to disturb will occur. During this age period children are too small to fight and too immature to express their sexual needs in reality. They live in a private and secret world in which they do and undo their isolation from full participation in the worlds of commerce and romance through fantasy. This can be achieved because humans alone have a capacity to abreact stresses and traumas through special symbols. These are the ludic symbols; described at length in other chapters. They serve *in loco personae* as objects to be involved in reliving, seeking vengeance, loving, and changing outcomes in memories of failure; all within the boundaries of fantasy. Ludic symbols are a subgroup of psychoanalytic symbols. They hold attention away from true affect laden problem memories, which are left to dwell as latent forces in the secret cellars of the mind. Ludic symbols are not simple holders of attention. They serve as partners in engagements which relive experiences that people seek to undo. Fantasy couple-hoods relive and abreact both humiliations and victories. Through active fantasy reliving, abreactive modifications of the remnants of experienced stresses can be achieved. A metaphor for this process is the physiological discharge of waste, called by Aristotle "catharsis'. The highest level of this function of the ludic symbol is achieved during the prelatency and the latency period. This special quality of ludic symbols supports education, delay of responses and development of identities, culture and religion during the latency years.

Adolescent growth and hormones provide real outlets through which experiences can be achieved, which outstrip the power of ludic symbols in fantasies. The ludic symbols of latency succumb to this shift in human potential. The process is called ludic demise. When the world of childhood is no longer there, their ludic potential for providing objects for abreaction and catharsis removed from the object world, are adopted in response to reality situations, which deny redress. Transference in therapy is an example.

Adults with talent use ludic symbols in poems, plays, and paintings of the sublime. Theistic preoccupations involve loved ludic equivalent entities, who help one to find forgiveness and abandon sorrow. Regression, to early physiologically expressed symbolic forms, produces cathartic discharge in the service of abreaction; a primitive form of ludic symbol. The case of Roy, presented in this chapter, illustrates this. Finally there is the recruitment of another person or thing as a ludic symbol to use for working through [abreaction, catharsis] of stress and conflict. The person must offer no logically valid potential for object discharge related to affect or conflict. When Roy (presented in this chapter,) treated me as though I were a fantasy based lesser subject person, he used me as a ludic symbol equivalent, in the transference.

THE BOY WHO WOULD BE KING

Roy Keiser came to therapy for an overt symptom. His symptom was encopresis, defined as stool retention with leakage. Roy had not been fully trained. He held back his stools, staining when he could no longer restrain himself. He had temper tantrums that disorganized him and the family. He could tolerate no frustration. He was four years old when therapy began.

When he was two years and nine months of age, a sister was born. There was a change in his personality, any progress in bowel control declined. He became obstinate, over-controlling, and very personalized in his selection of the time and place of defecation. From the day, his sister was born, he became very active, running from room to room. Increased activity is one of the outlets of a child with impaired or limited use of the symbolizing function. For three months he was persistently hyperactive, (started at 33 months). At 36 months, he was sent to nursery school where his pattern of over-control and retention of stool with leakage made him a somewhat odoriferous but "apparently toilet trained" three year old boy. Stool retention in school evaded detection by his teachers. At home, his soiled clothes told of episodes of loss of control. He could be put on the toilet without product only to lose control when his clothes were rearranged. There was no question that he could sense bowel fullness. At three and a half years of age, he had an impaction which was relieved by enema. This brought his problem to medical attention.

Megacolon, Hirschsprung's disease, disorders of colonic innervation, and absence of "anal wink"(sic) were ruled out and psychotherapy recommended.

He was weaned at 18 months. He sucked his thumb constantly. He had a distinct thumb sucker's bump proximal to the first right carpophalangeal joint. He had a security blanket which he carried with him continually when he was at home.

His mother was a tense self centered, money preoccupied woman. After discovering that my time for parent visits were subject to a fee, she shifted to frequent telephone calls. She tended to be overweight, which she kept under good control. She could cooperate in changes in patterns of parenting required for the therapy, such as limitation of severe punishments, disengagement from stimulating fecal cleansing activities, neutralizing of parental rage, reinforcement of symbolizing function (i.e. through reading fantasy material, inquiring about dreams, and discussions of enhanced cultural experiences such as movies and plays for children and encouragement of play with passively conceived Ludic Symbols.) The mother performed by rote with little grasp of dynamic balances within psychological ecologies, such as mutual influences and balances that characterize early child development and that inform therapeutic endeavors undertaken for people of that tender age.

Roy was a handsome, sturdy, very cooperative, verbal four and one half year old boy. In the evaluation of the symbolizing function in this toddler, it was found that his mental status was within normal limits except for deficiencies in fantasy forming functions. When asked about sleeping habits, he responded that "Sometimes I can't sleep - I think of having ice cream." He reports that he has never had a scary dream and doesn't make up stories.

When I began to introduce a ludic symbol, a Play-Doh soft long tube, he saw it as a snake. He could not put it into a story context or elaborate on the snake form. I concluded that he was capable of symbolic play, first seen in the 15 month old (See Piaget 1945), but not of producing true Ludic Psychoanalytic play symbols. There seemed to be a limit to his ability to create fantasy symbols and fantasies, which would have provided him with a more socially acceptable displaced outlet through which he could have resolved sibling rivalry conflicts.

We now digress to discuss the evaluation of the symbolizing function in the four year old. Note that above I said limited fantasy potential. I did not say that the symbolizing function was totally absent. When it comes to the evaluation of the viability of the symbolizing function in the service of fantasy in children, one must conceptualize the process within a context of an evolving complimentary series, remnants of each part of which may still be manifest after later stages have developed.

Relative health is determined by identifying the number and maturity of the symbolic forms available as well as the quality of the specific symbolic form that is utilized primarily in the production of manifest fantasy and behavior. If the reaction of the child aimed at adjustment to stress utilizes a manifest symbol selected from within the body boundary (in this regard see Sarnoff 1990), we deal with a symbolic form expressing reaction utilizing a body organ or product (a protosymbol). This is a precursor for what will in later life be called a Psychosomatic symptom, which is a truely evokative symbol with little in the way of a commmunicative pole. Were a child able to express his reaction through an external ludic (play object) symbol whose meaning is hidden from the therapist, we would say that we are dealing with a manifest symbol whose evocative pole is being emphasized; external and evoking, but not in the service of communication. At the more mature end of the complimentary series is the Psychoanalyic symbol used in the communicative mode. Here fantasy play contexts consist of symbol groupings which contain enough meaning detectable to the observer for the underlying (unconscious) meaning of the fantasy to be detected. With such symbols, eventually conscious discussion, interpretation and working through of the roots of represented problems can be introduced in preparation for the realities of adolescence. This is done best when interpretations will not destroy the function of the structure of latency. When his treatment began, Roy did not have the ability to form psychoanalytic symbols with ludic aspects. Roy's symbolic forms were limited to simple verbalizations, non-distortion dreaming and the use of body functions for power through regressed, evocative resolution of affect and conflict. This developmental cognitive impairment resulted in immature symbol formation, and permitted the persistence of fecal retention; a manifestation of anal phase power needs. A treatment strategy was devised to counter this. First the symbolizing function of the ego had to be improved so that the interaction between therapist and patient could be conducted in a zone that would permit self aware communication and interaction between the two. This step opened the way for the appearance of transference. Then the conflict and misunderstandings underlying the transference could be interpreted, identified and worked through. There follows a description of the application of this strategy in Roy's treatment.

TREATMENT

Roy's initial way of solving problems in sessions gave the impression of superior intelligence. He was neat and asked questions about the objects in the playroom. As he became more comfortable, however he began disorganized messing. Little was planned. There was also little in the way of organized fantasy. Attempts at painting which dominated his activities always resulted in mixed colors put on the paper in such large amounts that the table bore almost as much pigment as the paper. Early attempts at work with clay produced pizza, snakes without fantasy contexts, "duty" and a lot of clay on the floor and our shoes. If he dropped something, he asked or ordered me to pick it up, (a manifestation of characterological behavior). He ordered me to pick it up so often, that we resolved his demands by drawing a line on the linoleum playroom floor. Things that fell on my side, I picked up. Things that fell on his side, he picked up, sometimes.

There was poorly developed symbolizing function. His defensive resources were dominated by drive expression using primitive protosymbolic forms such as body parts and products. This shaped his behavior. When called upon in siuations of stress, these primitive defenses produced ego dissolution, increased messing, anxiety, and loss of control instead of the comfort to be derived from age appropriate fantasy formation. Mastery and discharge through the use of fantasy, which employs symbols sufficiently removed from the latent content to obscure meaning and associated affects, were not available to him. Because of this, I had recommended that the mother introduce the passive use of symbols through reading and story telling. In addition, I introduced activities during the sessions that were aimed at enhancement of cognition and symbolizing function. The clay moulding technique which is described in my book "Latency" (Sarnoff 1976) was introduced. I molded small clay figures of amorphous form asking him to guess what I was making. Whatever he guessed, I made. Once completed, these figures of his own creation, were permitted to dry. Once dried, the figures could be used to introduce the use of ludic symbols in fantasy. I asked questions which required the use of the figures in a story. I introduced use of his own symbols in a fantasy story.

In the twelfth month of treatment, I went out to welcome Roy in the waiting room. He rose from his seat slowly and having the sense that he had left something behind turned back for an instant, further slowing his progress toward the door of my office and playroom. His mother jumped up from her seat, and shoved him forward, pushing the base of his neck with such force that his head whip-lashed backward. As she pushed him, she said, "Go faster, you're wasting money." Two elements were added to the therapy as a result of her action. In a thrice, one could see an identification with mother's harsh controlling demands as one source of his characterological choice of bossiness. In addition, this situation provided an important inroad therapeutically. His mother's rejecting behavior turned his dependency needs toward a substitute object (the therapist). Removal of the primary object encouraged primary transference. Roy was so overwhelmed by feelings that he could not maintain his cold distance from me.

Tears streaming from his eyes, he cried to me, "Do you see that? Did you see what she did? She does that all the time." I had become his confidant. In turning to me, Roy had begun to live through or abreact his primary "transference wish" to be nurtured and cared for. In response to his mother's failure in this instance to give comfort he turned to the analyst as a substitute object. In this way he overcame some of his resistances and defense against relating dependently and began to undo the stilted nature of his object relations. This corrective object relationship experience apparently was followed by the mobilization of the communicative pole in the formation of symbols.

He marched from my consulting room into the play room. Tears gave way to anger. The anger too resolved as he began the first of a series of fantasies played out in the playroom. He took small gummed labels and began to past them on every toy in the room. On each he marked a value. He declared himself the owner of a store, he invited me to come in and buy. The play was awkward, without a medium of exchange. After a few sessions, this lack was responded to by the introduction of an industrial process that required my help because of its complexity. He organized the manufacture of coins to be used in his store. This included cardboard coins, gold foil covered coins, and even fabricated Olympic commemorative coins. A final stage in this play which lasted for months was the production of gold credit cards.

While working on the credit cards, he dropped a piece of gold foil paper on his side of the line.

He looked at me briefly and then curtly ordered me to pick up the scrap of paper. I pointed out its location. He cocked back his head, looked down his nose, and while pointing with haughty demeanor, commanded me to pick up the paper.

I looked straight back at him, while he continued his demands and bid me cooly to obey again and again. He had focused his characterological behavior in the therapy. He drove towards converting me as an object external to his body boundaries into a symbol of the stool he controlled at will.

Then I said "Who do you think you are?"

"I am a king." said he.

I was a little surprised. I realized at that moment that he had chosen a word, the knowledge of the meaning of which we could share to describe the sense of self that he demanded be recognized in his desperate need to undo the inferiority and the narcissistic vulnerability that formed the core of his self image. This demand aimed at me was a form of transference. Finding a name (KING) could make it possible for us to share, look at, discuss, come back to, and make this barely conscious concept that had been used as defense available to the system consciousness. McClure (1991) has described how "Naming something makes it stand out more clearly from the surrounding background." (p110) Luria (1968) pp 120-123, speaks of "the forms of reflection which are realized through speech". And Sachs, (1989) speaks of "the acquisition of conceptualizing and systematizing power with language." (p43) In a

person who is fearful of harm from loved ones, some
concepts have too much affect to be spelled out
in words. In these cases symbolic substitutes such
as the therapist are invoked, who are sufficiently
removed from the original to hide meaning. The more
fearful or autistic the child, the less are these
symbols used in a communicative mode. Interpretation
can bring their true meaning into consciousness.

Insight and the possibility of working through
occurred when we shared the aftermath of the reality
situation in the waiting room. At that point Roy
was able to represent drives through symbols that
though masked had a communicative aspect that
could be used for interpretation and expansion of
consciousness to include explanations of previously
inexplicable transference behavior.

In response to his declaration that he was a king, my
thoughts dwelled on the possibility of approaching
insight through the symbol he had introduced (a
King). He needed to be a king, I thought because
he felt so unimportant. I suspected that pursuit
of the king symbolism could provide knowledge
with enough distance to be psychotherapeutically
workable. However it soon became clear that such
working through would have to wait for another
day for he began to cut a long strip of cardboard
creating a saw-toothed edge. He glued gold paper to
the cardboard and then pasted on brightly colored
play-doh "jewels". He twisted the strip into a loop
large enough to circle his head and then, placing
it upon his brow, marked the end of the session by

marching proudly from the room wearing a symbol of the king, a Golden Crown.

I was confronted with an enigma. To interpret his royal presumption might result in leaving him defenseless, in terror, and depressed. I remembered the South African proverb that admonished, "Don't take anything of value from a man, unless you can give him something of value in return."

In subsequent sessions, we pursued his idea that he was a king. Logically he could not be a king because a king's father is always a king. He had got the concept of king from the fairy tale books his parents had read to him and in his experience, kings were the sons of kings. He was easily able to put aside nameing himself a king. The underlying concept needed more attention. I pointed out the linkage of his kingship to his encopresis. I said, "When you thought you were a king, you could make a duty any place you want to". "And anytime I want to", said he. From that session forth his encopretic witholding came under control.

This insight was not enough to modify his character traits. There was left to be worked through the reason that he needed to feel he was something special with special rules like a king. We were embarked on an investigation of his sense of humiliation when scolded by his mother and his feeling that money was more important to her than he was. He also had feelings of jealousy for his sibling who was seen to be held as more valuable than he. The working through of these important areas were averted when his mother, encouraged by the subsidence of the encopresis and with a lack of psychological mindedness that caused her to see treatment results as the product of a sort of magic, withdrew the child from treatment.

Discussion of the "Boy Who Would Be King"

Verbal Representation and Mental Content in the Toddler

Roy's anal sadistic drives were expressed through body organ based protosymbols when he came to treatment and so were not available at first to an understanding, which could be productive of verbal interpretation and influence.

A transition from affecto-motor memory to verbal concept memory, which Roy had only partially completed before he came for therapy left much that was encoded in the affectomotor memory system and unavailable to the awareness system to which psychotherapy is geared. That awareness system detects verbalizations primarily. Not every event or experience in the child's world finds a word. Roy was slow in this area, especially when it came to the cushioning effect of the symbolizing function, which makes representation possible, albeit in masked form. Roy had no words for what his anger expressed or meant to him, when he started therapy. This is a form of repression that works by exclusion through an absence of a conduit to verbally organized consciousness. (Schachtel 1949). Cognitive structures for use in producing symbolic or verbal communication were not yet adequately mature in Roy, for utilization. Rather than use symbols and

fantasies, in response to his mother's ease to anger
and the birth of a sib, Roy's compensatory narcissism
generated physiological expression. Messing, bowel
with-holding, and demanding controlling behavior
(transference) in the therapy.

Therapeutic goals included verbalized insight.
This required techniques to encourage more mature
symbolic forms. This goal was achieved through the
introduction of psychoanalytic symbols using words
and concepts derived from the zone of experience
beyond the boundary of the self. This raised the
level of instinctual expression to the point at
which communication and interpretation became
possible. The verbalization and identification of an
age available form of transference were realized.
Developmentally, the acquisition of the capacity to
utilize psychoanalytic symbols in a communicative
mode is a turning point with many implications.
The development of latency with its importance
for civilization begins. The introduction of
communicative symbols and words to interpret them
enhance verbalized insight and aid in the resolution
of conflict. Note that the budding structure of
latency was not approached with interpretation aimed
at minimizing it. The interpretations dealt with
the expression of power needs that were interfering
with the advent of latency function and defenses.

When early infantile wishes or the memory residua
of trauma can be symbolized communicatively, speech
can be used in resolving transference. This entails
working through of and disenabling of the contents
of the core and masturbation fantasies which are the

precursors of adult transferences, characterology,
fate neuroses and neurotic symptoms. Communicative
discharge and confrontation are enabled by
the development of speech and the evolving of
decipherable cryptic symbols. These permit the
organization and expression of fantasy informed
infantile sexual wishes on increasingly more mature,
socially acceptable and sublimated levels. Organ
protosymbols sidetrack this trend. The symbols are
too primitive and evocative Adjustment is interfered
with as in the case of Roy whose use of control of
his stools expressed his anger and control needs
and defied his mother. Psychoanalytic symbols in the
communicative mode serve compromise formation and
permit discharge under more socialized conditions.
Through the interpretation of such symbols,
otherwise irretrievable transferences based on early
infantile wishes or the memory residua of trauma
can be converted from that, which is only acted or
felt to that, which can be expressed in symbols.
which can be interpreted into verbal concepts that
can be worked through or associated to, confronted,
or challenged.

In Roy's case, a developmental step in symbol
usage was introduced to the therapy so that
interpretation of transference behavior could
bring unconscious motivation into consciousness.
Verbalization in children enhances the working
through of and disenabling of contents that are
destined to underlie transference wishes in adults.
Communicative discharge and confrontation followed
upon the development of speech and the evolving
of decipherable cryptic symbols. This permits the

organization and expression of infantile sexual wish informed fantasy, which can be interpreted in child therapy. This results in controlled reparative mastery, working through and the confrontation of the "sense of reality" by "reality testing".

The effective interpretation of transference results in a self reflective awareness. This awareness places the content of past events and future effects, attitudes, and behavior within reach during the therapy session. The patient expands his consciousness creating a lucid image by expanding the view he has of himself to include that which had formerly been repressed or left unconscious. In this way, the person becomes aware of behavior and motivation, and can recognize that which makes the behavior inappropriate. This brings into focus, with the therapist's help, reasons for stopping the behavior.

The evolution of consciousness is the evolution of self reflexive verbal thought. This should be differentiated from other awarenesses such as awareness of reflex signals and the responses and awareness that accompany semi-facultative "automatic" responses that have been learned or have become second nature as in dancing or athletics.

A major transition in a child's awareness occurs when word memory representing abstract concepts become associated with percepts and affects and other experiences of the moment that had previously only called for reflex responses. Words that represent abstractions can be recalled and remembered. Such recall of abstractions opens the way to past and future, and expands awareness to encompass a view of life that adds insight and a sustained longitudinal history of meaning to experience. The role of interpretation is to expand this memory resonance.

THE LATENCY LINKED CYCLE OF THE LUDIC SYMBOL

THERAPEUTIC ENTRÉE POINTS WITH CHILDREN AT PLAY

The world of the latency age child holds him distant from drive gratifying interactions with reality. In place of real objects, the child turns to toys, songs, and found object as symbolic replacements. These choices are tuned to the child's maturation, development and growth.

During the latency years, there is a cycle of change involving ludic symbols. The cycle may be completed in a flash or take years to unfold. The cycle begins with the child's selection of the object to be used as a symbol. Usually this object is of three dimensions and has weight. It is selected from toys in the playroom. This is followed by a trial period to see if it will work to both conceal and reveal a latent content in memory. (Piaget 1945) Sometimes the toy is rejected and replaced with a more appropriate object. Inherent in the selection process is an aspect that can be put to use by a child therapist. The chosen toy can be introduced by the therapist. Like an interpretation made to an adult patient the suggested ludic symbol can be chosen for its ability to enhance the already present direction of the child's free association. In this way appropriate abreactive fantasies with potential affect resolution can be encouraged. The toy can be retained in a personal bin so that each future session retains the theme. If no suitable toy is available, images can be drawn or molded for use as puppets that elaborate fantasy. The child's own images can be used, including elements from dreams drawn and cut out for that purpose. Ludic symbols can be used to achieve reparative mastery through fantasy.

The cycle comes to an end, when the child grows, and reality offers satisfaction as ludic symbols dwindle. The transition from objects in fantasy to reality objects characterizes the symbols of the dwindling ludic fantasy. The therapist is there to discuss and work through the child's finding of a root in reality for himself. His intervention may be concrete or abstract depending on the child's level of cognition. The end of the cycle offers the therapist a portal of entry into the growing personality of the child.

UNIT SIX

TERMINATION

TERMINATION

THE CRITERIA FOR DECIDING TO TERMINATE THERAPY IN DYNAMIC CHILD PSYCHOTHERAPY ARE-

1. The presenting problem has been resolved.

2. Access to motor expression for fantasy based motivations is within age acceptable bounds.

3. The child's academic and social activities reflect a reality focus appropriate to his age.

4. The child's progression in development reflects a stage and rate that is commensurate with that of successful peers.

5. Further therapeutic work will produce progress that age appropriate natural development could provide as well.

6. An awareness of reality through age/phase appropriate shared consciousness has been achieved.

7. Development of symbol formation should be age appropriate.

Problems that may be Encountered During Termination

<u>Aberrant symbolic interpretations of reality</u> by children are not pathological if they conform to cultural, religious, or political norms. Too much conformity to beliefs that are potentially dangerous and are not limited by mature judgment may lead to perilous behavior, If that is so, adult supervision should be suggested to limit the child. This should not interdict termination.

<u>The therapist becomes more and more a love object in the termination phase.</u> One must beware that the patient in this phase may find a reality person to love; shift her attention to the new object; lose interest in the therapist; and drop out of treatment. (a termination phenomenon called "Removal" by Annie Reich.)

<u>The reappearance of original symptoms</u> is a frequent occurrence during termination. This may be interpreted to be a wish to continue treatment.

<u>A sense of passivity in the child intensifies.</u> The nature of childhood dictates a passive subjugated role in society. The preschool child asks, "Who is the boss of me?"). In late _latency,_ there is resentment resulting from being "half the size of anyone else and not (having) a dime to (one's) name") Where termination is really a forced interruption that serves the personal needs of the therapist or the parents, this sense of passivity is strengthened in the child. The child may resent decisions made without his input. One should be on the alert for

the presence of this situation and associated reactions and manipulations by the child in respect
to this situation. Techniques, which permit the
child to join in the decision to terminate, should
be introduced. For instance permitting the child
to join in the decision to terminate, and in the
selection of the date of termination, can counter
the sense of passivity.

THE TECHNIQUE of TERMINATION

Once it has been determined through conference
between the parents and the therapist that goals
originally set are near resolution, the child is
asked if there are problems for which he feels he
needs further help. If there are no such problems,
a date is set to set an initial date for deciding
to end therapy. The termination date chosen then
may be put off repeatedly or finalized, determined
by the child's heightened awareness and sustained
progress in the therapy sessions.

Sessions, during termination, are not spent waiting.
Intensification of therapeutic activity marks the
period. Feelings about the departing therapist
energize fantasies. These psychological *reactions*
can be mined therapeutically. For instance loss
of the therapist as love object may threaten the
patient. The child who is threatened by homoerotic
feelings may become acutely uncomfortable when
he perceives warm feelings for a therapist of the
same sex. It is necessary to point out to such a
child that the feelings he has for the departing
therapist are the expected products of working with

a person over a prolonged period. The relationship can be likened to that between father and son. As such, the homoerotic implications of the feelings can be resolved by an interaction, which involves a blurring of roles and self boundaries such as occurs after talking about the therapist's life realities. This provides a basis for internalizing elements of the therapist, which obviates the sense of loss.

THE SEVEN PHASES IN THE MATURATION OF AWARENESS

FOR TERMINATION TO BE CONSIDERED,
A RESHAPING OF AWARENESS INTO A PHASE
APPROPRIATE KIND OF CONSCIOUSNESS,
RESULTING FROM THE MATURATION OF
SYMBOLIZATION, SHOULD BE PRESENT.

PHASE ONE

Information in regard to phase one (birth to 24 months) does not apply directly to termination. It is presented because that, which is past is prologue.

The term consciousness, in early phase one, refers to awareness before ever strengthening repression-influenced symbolization develops. Attention and immediate response to sensations is syncretic and "conscious" in the phase one new-born child. These protagonists part company, when displacement [at 2 1/2yrs]. and repression [at 4yrs] enable delay of response to inputs; providing time to permit experience, drives and the personality needs of the child to influence the selection of responses.

Internal sensations dominate in phase one. This arrangement provides a paradigm for internal sources in later years to shape conscious awareness based on neurotic motivations and distortions derived from feelings and memories independent of the current world.

Add varying intensity of drives, as the child grows, reflections of experience, acquired wisdom, and the plangent influences of brain hormone and chemical changes to the mix of influences on the child's thinking. These are the phase related factors, which overwhelm the influence of reality in a child's thinking, as he passes on the way to maturity, through the phases described below.

It is during late phase one (18 to 24 months) that the first ascents from basic animal awareness coupled with immediate reflex responses, begin to make way for the later six stages of childhood human conscious awareness. The stages of conscious awareness are built around ascent from reflex to awareness and response informed by memory. A time gap opens between input and response [disjuncture] through which slip shaping influences such as past experience, judgment, and wisdom that alter responses in the service of self preservation, and the future.

PHASE TWO

During phase two, primitive sustained, conscious awareness is reshaped by symbolization. Weak repression truncates perception and shapes memory, As a result accurate subsequent interpretation of reality can be impaired. Dynamic psychotherapy first becomes possible. A phase two (26 months to 4 years) therapy case follows.

Little Jan was brought for therapy by parents whose vacation at the beach was impaired by their twenty-six month old child's strongly felt fear of sea-weed. She expressed her fear freely, in phrasing that implied that everyone must know what she was talking about. When she was asked whom she was angry at, for sea-weed doesn't get angry, but little girls do, she directed her attention to complaints about her mother, who left her alone afternoon and night in the care of a strange baby sitter. The mother was encouraged to reorganize her schedule. The child returned the seaweed to its role as a pale agent in the environment. A dynamically influenced modification in the family system supported the insight gained through symbolized psychotherapeutic interpretive questioning

The earliest age at which insight oriented psychotherapy can be applied as treatment for mental pathology is twenty-six months. This timing is based on clinical observations and the researches of Jean Piaget. The underlying process is a maturation of a weak capacity to repress that supports the creation of symbols with hidden meanings. Such repression is produced through a

displacement of the attention of the child away from
suppressed anger, which had originally been meant
for a loved one, to the aggressive potential, (i.e.
something imagined - projected) of something in
the environment. Attention is diverted from affect
and its associated objects or memories., These
elements are, as a result, deserted: left to persist
in a gelid Gehenna (*underworld*), which is unknown
(*UNBEWUSST*) to conscious awareness.

TREATMENT- The predominant pathological symptoms of
phase two are: phobia for plants or interpretations
of new perceptions as hostile, while the child
is under stress. The repression that produces
these symptoms is easily disrupted. Attention is
shaped into a consciousness in which perception
and memory is distorted. Awareness of affect laden
concepts is truncated, leaving only symbolic forms
(countercathexes) available to consciousness (i.e
phobic objects such as seaweed) These manifest
remnants of total experience support exclusion by
repression. Between two and a half and four years
repression is weak. Direct discussion with the child
to identify the anger causing situation is possible.
This should be followed by advice to caretakers
about reorganizing the family system.

PHASE THREE

Prelatency

3 ½ years to 5 yrs of age

Normally at this age, there is only fair reality
testing with a poor sense of reality. As a result,

internal conflicts can be resolved through a sense of reality that makes of fantasy more than play. They are therefore ideal candidates for play therapy. Reality can and should be interpreted during therapy.

Play (LUDIC) symbols, described as first appearing at this age by Piaget, perform the same role in resolving stress and conflict resolution as do the dream symbols that process irrational thinking and motivation during adult REM sleep.

In phase three, the repression involved in the production of symbols is strengthened, for reality offers a weak seat in which attention can rest before it is altered into a consciousness dominated by preconceptions [memory and prior symbolizations]. Easily distorted interpretation of the world (physis) based on prior experience and learning is set up, often for life. Such symbolization may serve to provide an illusion of knowledge. This is a mastery skill to be used throughout life in defending against new perceptions and inputs regarding religion, sports, regard for parental points of view, and politics, as well as a means of distracting the child from an uncomfortable urge, fantasy or memory.

Aberrant symbolic interpretations of reality by children is not necessarily pathological at this age. Prior education can play a large part. For example: A suburban father and his almost 5 year-old son embarked for the city to see the circus. Leaving the car of a friend in a place far from the circus venue, the father led his son by hand into a New York City Subway station. Proudly the boy announced, "This is a cave. Mommy read me a story about caves." At a level below the street and one flight of steps above the tracks, the boy grasped his father's hand more tightly, in response to the sound of an express train's roar as it tore through the station. "Are you all right?" asked the father. "I think that's a dragon", was the reply. "No, That's a train. You'll soon see." said the father. Before the father could stop speaking, the loud roar, of a stopping train, drowned out his words. Passengers rushed up the stairs and proceeded pell-mell to the exit to the street. The boy pulled his hand free and joined the maddening crowd. The father rushed after. Grabbing his son's hand, he demanded, "What are you thinking?" The boy replied, "If this isn't a cave and that's not a dragon, why are all those people running?"

PHASE FOUR-

-Early Latency (1) 6 - 8 1/2 yrs.-

In phase four (6 to 8 ½ years), sources of the child's view of himself shift from the family to school peers and teachers. Children become defiant of parents as they take on the attitudes of teachers and peers in developing a self image independent of parental influence.

Example:

"Beaming, the mother said "Bubala it's your first day of school. Already you're six years old and you're gonna make us so proud. I'm so proud of you

Bubala. Here comes the bus. Go! Make us proud!" "Yes mamma." said the boy.

"Proud, Bubala, proud."

"Yes, yes.", said the boy

Hours later, the boy returned. He entered the home slowly.

Undeterred by his truculent mood, the mother demanded. "So what did you learn today Bubala?" The boy seemed to tremble, his voice uncertain.

"So what did you learn?"

"I learned."

"Yes"

"I LEARNED,... I learned... 'My name is Irving."

Maturation of the symbolizing function, in early latency, is the result of the strengthening of repression that develops at 48 months: resulting from denial of inner states and denial supporting projection to the world, which shapes the form of manifest (consciously experienced) symbols. Truncation of potential conscious memory content as a result of symbolization that alters perception, memory, abstract hopes and expectations, change the organization of the child's image of the world and the future. Repression supporting symbols distort reality. They enhance suppression of the influence of experience and memory during the years 6 to 12 [latency]. These symbols are not transparent. They do not give way to interpretation. This presages the impaired sense of reality function sometime found later as a part of mature consciousness.

Repression based symbols and associated dream like fantasy play are the primary defenses of latency; a time when the child is passive and physically helpless, when confronting the world.

The therapist should emphasize playing and symbols in the treatment of the latency age child and not analyze them. Interpret away the symbols and the child will be overwhelmed by anxiety. Beware of being asked to medicate a child whose anxiety is a product of attempting to interpret away the curtain of symbols, which hold painful memories and impossible goals out of awareness. The patient may be calmed by medication; but resolution of conflict and impulse through fantasy and play may be bypassed, leaving a pathological personality-radical in place: to influence adult character.

PHASES FIVE and SIX

Phase five - Late latency (2)

From 8 ½, (WHEN PLAY SYMBOLS BEGIN

GRADUALLY TO WEAKEN IN THEIR

ABILITY TO PROCESS TENSION AND

TRAUMA)

To 11, (WHEN THE PATIENT MOVES INTO

THE TALKING ROOM AND ABSTRACT PROVERB

INTERPRETATION IS POSSIBLE)

In phase five (late latency), the ability of repression influenced symbols to serve drive discharge wanes and reality elements become the symbolic forms that include for instance the therapist in the fantasies that infuse transference during termination.

In PHASE SIX – Late latency through early adolescence (11 years to 13 years) there is an intensification of the tilt to realistic external elements as the source of manifest symbolic forms. This shift leads eventually to a conversion of latency age conscious fantasy into a tool for future planning. In the termination phase, the therapist becomes more and more the love object. One must beware that the patient in this phase may find a reality person to love; shift her attention to the new object; lose interest in the therapist; and drop out of treatment. (a termination phenomenon called "Removal".)

In the PHASE SEVEN shift, there is a shift from play [ludic] symbols to humanoid and human figures, as a source of objects to love. This can result in a termination love transference, characterized by the late-latency-early adolescent tilt of the direction of manifest symbol selection toward choosing countercathectic external reality inputs. Such symbols support repression, which binds the excited energies of emotion. If effective, this frees the mind to work in reality and avoid pursuing that which is physically not possible.

There is a downside to this. As physical possibility increases with growth and fantasy objects are replaced by reality objects, heightened over--stimulation by lovers can overwhelm the capacity of repression oriented symbols to handle emotional stress. This can result in diminution of the neutral energies requiring for learning activities and may introduce difficulty in keeping junior high school students focused on work.

A bright side to this process is the development of the ability to fall in love - defined as an increased capacity to experience the world as a place to share with others. This is part of the age enhanced process of turning toward reality in search of objects for drive expression. The end product of this process <a biologically driven march of developmental events> is the attainment of a relationship with a partner for procreative sex, which is dominated by mutual justice.

PHASE SEVEN

15 Years to Adulthood

Adolescence ends with adult object choice in which justice is combined with passion and the needs of the partner influence the behavior of the lover.

Conscious fantasy symbols no longer serve as supporters of repression. They are replaced with simple representations: environmental elements that can be integrated into realistic future planning.

INTERMINABLE CHILD THERAPY

Therapeutic success can be sabotaged by persistent psychopathogenic parental pessimism directed at the patient. I call such parents "crushers". The treatment situation in these cases can come to an end, but the termination criteria may not be satisfied. A child, who was brought to me for therapy in late latency had such a parent. His father described his feelings about his child as beloved excrement. Such denigrating parenting lowers the self image of a child. Should the effect of such whimsical fantasies not pass, its constant renewal could undermine therapeutic gain, and contribute to adult character.

UNIT SEVEN -

LITERATURE

LITERATURE > BIOGRAPHY > AUTOBIOGRAPHY ARE AN IMITATION OF LIFE

Goethe's Child Psychiatry Time Capsule

jds — In other sections of this book you refer to "informed perception". What is implied by this concept is that one sees what he is prepared to see by training and prior experience. Has psychoanalytic understanding distorted and informed our perception of childhood mental illness, or has a psychopathological entity, formed and influenced by unconscious fantasy and motivation, escaped notice till now?,

CAS

The latter concept is correct. The informed perceptions that underlay the understanding of mental illness throughout history have been legion. The idea of unconscious motivation underlying neurosis is of recent origin.

Many theories have supported many therapies. Fear
of spirit intrusions supported therapeutic efforts
to expel the spirits or children were encouraged to
bear the pressure of mythic entities, who intruded
on them in the night. Demoniacal possession was
understood to be related to seduction by the
devil, and treated by extirpation or punishable
by immolation. The development of other theories
was precluded, and a dynamic unconscious influence
was excluded from the list. Words, to describe the
influence of a dynamic unconscious on behavior, were
not available before 1895. The concept of a dynamic
unconscious with repressed content, and impelled
to awareness by drives, could not be formulated.
The concept of a dynamic influence of unconscious
motivation and affect charged fantasy on symptoms
and behavior was beyond reach. Without concepts
in words to be shared between investigators in
support of exploration, research was impossible.
The influence of novelists such as George Eliot
and Wilkie Collins, who referred to "unconscious"
without dynamic factors, did not advance theory.
Without concepts put into written words to be shared
with future historians, there could not have been
left a record of the existence of psychopathology
as we know it. This would make an answer to your
question impossible. Gaining access to a view into
the nursery of hundreds of years ago, in search of
concepts and entities for which recording minds had
no words, seems beyond reach. How could one know?
Find a record that gives a "life beyond life" to the
experiences of a eighteenth century troubled child.

One exists. A great writer, Goethe, wrote a retrospective study of his emotional life. He has left us a "time capsule" with descriptions of the psychopathology that appeared during the phases of his life. Written when he was 70 years old, it is called "Dichtung und Wahrheit" ("Truth and Fiction Relating to My Life" Kindle Loc 12). A study of his childhood pathology tells us that signs and symptoms have not changed. Study of the appearance of fear fantasies, identities and moods in his adult literary works tell us of retention of conflicts over time, locked through life in his unconscious. Study of the impact of childhood themes on his mature literary works, makes it possible to trace the dynamic influence of childhood fears and fantasies, on adult pathology and poetry.

The existence of childhood pathology (night fears, fear of heights, and projection) is described by Goethe in writings that predate the addition to informed perception of dynamic theory.

Childhood Pathology, And Moods Night Fears

Goethe in early childhood feared darkness and dreaded night creatures that would harm him. He reported the situation thus-

Goethe KINDLE Loc 539

"The old, many-cornered, and gloomy arrangement of the house was, moreover adapted to awaken dread and terror in childish minds. Unfortunately, too, the principle of discipline, that young persons should

be early deprive of all fear for the awful and
invisible, and accustomed to the terrible, still
prevailed. We children, therefore were compelled to
sleep alone; and when we found this impossible and
softly slid from our beds, to seek the society of
servants and maids, our father, with his dressing
gown turned inside out, which disguised him
sufficiently for the purpose, placed himself in the
way, and frightened us back to our resting places.
The evil effect of which anyone may imagine. How is
he who is encompassed with a double terror to be
emancipated from fear? My mother, always cheerful
and gay, and willing to render others so, discovered
a much better pedagogical expedient. She managed
to gain her ends with rewards. Peaches. Promised
each morning. The promise of which overcame our
fears during the night. In this way she succeeded
and both parties were satisfied."

How old was Goethe then? In his comments on "Dichtung
und Wahrheit" Freud (1925) placed these events before
four years of age (p 147). This would place the night
fears at a point where symbolic representation
is possible. (beyond two and a half years). Fear
of the dark was a developmental possibility once
repression could occur (four years) and be sustained
through displacement and symbolization and could be
expressed through night fears. The content of the
fears is not described. Later manifestations support
the following themes: projection of aggression in
response to a rigid father, preoccupation with the
devil and the afterlife, fear of becoming a stolen
child, and being more vulnerable in darkness.

Klopstock in the Nursery

How could the Goethe children know enough to fear
that a dark agent would come in the night and harm
them? Children died. Children disappeared. Could
it be that they had experienced the death of their
siblings? No. There were four siblings all born
after Goethe was 6 years old. The four, who died,
died after Goethe was ten years old. The timing
isn't right.

It is known that Goethe's sister, Cornelia, who was
a year and a half younger than Goethe participated
with him in puppet shows, toy theatres, and plays,
encouraged by their mother. The father was stern
and not given to sympathy. He married at thirty-
seven. The mother was sympathetic, warm, and apt
to take the children's side. She knew that her
husband abhorred the bright style of Klopstock.
In spite of this, she bought a small volume of
Kopstock's Messiah (1748) and carried it hidden in
her pocket. She read tales of the devil, and hell
from it to the children. They knew of places to
which stolen children could be taken. At one time
the sister, setting aside the requirement that the
children speak low in the presence of their father,
began to shout lines from Klopstock's Messiah. Her
capacity to speak words makes her older than 2½.
and Wilhelm at least four. Her loud words were heard
by the barber who was ministering to the father.
He spilled fluid on the father. The father banished
Klopstock from the nursery. Too late, a seed had
been imbedded in the children's memories. Over the
years branches growing from that seed were there

to manifest themselves in night fears, neuroses, "Faust", "The Erlenkoenig", and Mignon.

LATENCY: THE LONGING HEART (sehnsucht hertz)

In his life and writings there was a feeling of solitude, a sense of vague longing, awe implanted by nature, the pressure of the too gloomy and powerful. They become stronger when under stress. He describes the first flowering of these feelings in the following.

Goethe KINDLE Loc. 532

"On the second floor was a room, which was called the garden-room, because they had there endeavored to supply the want of a garden by means of a few plants placed before the windows. As I grew older, it was there that I made my favorite, not melancholy. but somewhat sentimental retreat. In the summer season I commonly learned my lessons there, and watched the thunderstorms. …I saw the neighbors...children… gardens (I) could hear the bowls rolling and the ninepins dropping, It early excited in me a feeling of solitude, and a sense of vague longing resulting from it which conspired with the seriousness and, exerted its influence at so early an age, and showed itself more distinctly in after-years.

He experienced "…the pressure of the too gloomy and powerful, which continued to rule … within (him)"

These feelings appear in the personalities of many of the protagonists of his writings.

ADOLESCENCE - CAUGHT BY A FAULTY
RECOMMENDATION

Kindle loc. 3193 etseq.

Leaving childhood behind, Goethe reached out to new friends and to Gretchen, with whom he fell in love. The friends led him astray. They sought his recommendation to a position of some merit for a young man well recognized as of poor character. The situation went badly. A judicial inquiry explored Goethe's role. He was interrogated and confined to his home. Gretchen left town after declaring their relationship had been that of a caretaker to a child. He was exonerated. Yet he had been involved, and been sequestered. In describing his then emotional state, Goethe recalled depression, self destructive ideation, grief, and passionate solitude. A melancholy condition of infinite yearning, and raving and lassitude persisted. He sought to contain these feelings with focusing on preparation for his forthcoming departure for the university. He sought to banish his depression by activity. There remained a paranoid sense that in the market place "the most indifferent glances annoyed him". "hypochondriasis" took much of his attention.. He resolved these residua by leaving the agora for the woods. (Kindle loc. 3368) Paranoid preoccupations and low mood were less cathected, when he left for college in Freibourg where he took up with a group of students who devoted themselves to finding faults in others.

TUBERCULOSIS

After three years of university training, Goethe
experienced a massive bleeding episode during
the night. His recovery period lasted one and a
half years. Encoded in memory, this experience is
recalled in "Wilhelm Meister" (1795-6) in Book Six
of Volume Two. "Confessions of a Beautiful Soul" A
woman speaks. "I had a hemorrhage at the start of
my eighth year." And "During the nine months that
I was confines to bed…" (Page 135) there appeared
remembered elements; described in the Goethe quote
from "Wilhelm Meister" (see below) in which Art was
shaped by memory. Though "The song is ended, the
memory lingers on."

(Goethe kindle loc 4914)

"One night, I awoke with a violent hemorrhage, and
had just strength and presence of mind enough to
awaken my next-room neighbor [a doctor was called]…
For many days I wavered between life and death."
"…during that eruption, a tumor had formed on the
left side of the neck." According to Jensen (2015)
Goethe was afflicted with tuberculosis requiring two
years convalescence. There had been lung caseation,
cavitation, invasion of an artery and a scrofulous
involvement of a lymph gland in the neck. In my
early medical career, I worked in a tuberculosis
hospital; providing me with an ability to describe
this pathology, and confirm this diagnosis. Goethe
left school and returned to his home. A rest cure
of over a year was appropriate at the time. His
mother was supportive, his sister less so and his
father distant. In his father's presence, he had

to be "on one's guard … against hypochondriacal expressions, because (the father) … could then become passionate and bitter." Once recovered, Goethe, under pressure from his father, went to Law School in Strasburg where his interests strayed from the law to poetry and writing. Much of his time was devoted to addressing multiple psychological symptoms, such as fear of heights, treated with behavior modification. [kindle 5566] He arrived in Strasburg with an irritability persisting from his recent physiological brush with death.

As he put it -

Goethe KINDLE Loc 5565

"I was then in a state of health which furthered me sufficiently in all that I would and should undertake; only there was a certain irritability left behind, which did not always let me be in equilibrium. A loud sound was disagreeable to me, diseased objects awakened in me loathing and horror. But I was especially troubled with a giddiness, which came over me every time I looked down from a height. All these infirmities I tried to remedy, and, indeed, as I wished to lose no time, in a somewhat violent way. In the evening, when they beat the tattoo, I went near the multitude of drums, the powerful rolling and beating of which might have made one's heart burst in one's bosom. All alone I ascended the highest pinnacle of the minster spire, and sat in what is called the neck, under the nob or crown, for a quarter of an hour, before I would venture to step out again into the open air, where, standing upon a platform scarce an ell square, without any particular holding, one sees the boundless prospect before; while the nearest objects and ornaments conceal the church, and every thing upon and above which one stands. It is exactly as if one saw one's self carried up into the air in a balloon. Such troublesome and painful sensations I repeated until the impression became quite indifferent to me; and I have since then derived great advantage."

This description reflects the late eighteenth century approach to anxiety associated symptoms of an emotional disorder. This was the use of repeated exposure to the objects feared aimed at achieving desensitization. Goethe applied this technique to more general areas of abhorrence,

In his words 'Anatomy, also, was of double value to me, as it taught me to endure the most repulsive sights, while I satisfied my thirst for knowledge. And thus I also attended the clinical course of the elder Dr. Ehrmann, as well as the lectures of his son on obstetrics, with the double view of becoming acquainted with all conditions, and of freeing myself from all apprehension as to repulsive things. And I have actually succeeded so far, that nothing of this kind could ever put me out of my self-possession. But I endeavored to harden myself, not only against these impressions on the senses, but also against the infections of the imagination. The awful and shuddering impressions of the darkness in churchyards, solitary places, churches, and chapels by night, and whatever may be connected with them, I contrived to render likewise indifferent; and in this, also, I went so far that day and night, and every locality, were quite the same to me: so that even when, in later times, a desire came over me once more to feel in such scenes the pleasing shudder of youth, I could hardly compel this, in any degree, by calling up the strangest and most fearful image."

It should be noted that this was the then current psychiatric treatment approach. His father had used a similar suppressive approach in dealing with his children's night fears.

After one and a half years Goethe took and failed his final exams. Instead of a doctorate in law, he was given a license to practice law. He went then to Weimar to observe the working of law courts there. Befriended by the young Duke of Weimar, he became a diplomat, a "von" and began to devote himself to poetry and literature. He wrote "Werther" and "Gotz". Fame followed. By this time, Goethe was in his mid-twenties. Thenceforth there are no available reports relating to long periods of inanition or neurotic fears or serious emotional episodes. Latent fantasies instead found form in his writings.

LATENT NEUROTIC FANTASY THEMES THAT APPEAR IN GOETHE'S WRITINGS

Goethe, as a child had a tendency, as do other children, to distort reality to conform to the influence of his own intruding and affect charged unconscious entities. In early childhood he was troubled by fears in darkness and initial feelings of loneliness and despair. In adult life fantasies and feelings and inappropriate affects were dealt with differently. Instead of the neurotic decompensations of childhood there appeared in dealing with conflict a maneuver, from which Goethe could not deviate. Dominating his adjustment to everything was the creation of an image or a poem, often in the form of a symbol based sublimation; a work of art. This technique helped resolve conflict through providing some certain understanding within himself that might both rectify his concepts of the nature of external things that his informed perception had interpreted to be stressful, and set his mind at rest about them.

In his own words, Goethe said,

"And thus began that tendency from which I could not deviate my whole life through; namely the tendency to turn into an image, into a poem everything that delighted or troubled me, or otherwise occupied me and to come to some certain understanding within myself about it, that I might both rectify my concepts of external things, and set my mind at rest about them"

In childhood troubling memories that are imbedded rise to consciousness in the form of intermittent fears and moods. They can be processed, understood, and reparatively mastered or worked through during child therapy sessions. In adulthood, unconscious fantasies, can be resolved through sublimations; art, written projects, theatre, music, play and psychotherapy. Other maneuvers used by Goethe for the avoidance of conflict and stressful situations were marriage avoidance, and extended travel.

WORKING THROUGH USING FANTASY AND PLAY IN CHILD THERAPY

SUBLIMATION AS DEFENSE

Conversion of a percept into a concept in memory associated with an affect adds a distressing irritant to unconscious content. Such irritants attract conscious awareness, Conscious emergence of the representation requires that it be modified by displacement, projection, or symbolization, sufficiently so that overwhelming of the experiencing self [consciousness] does not take place. Mastery in the face of this possibility requires. sublimation and working through using displaced or symbolized manifestations of the troubling element. Goethe, upon leaving home and school in his mid twenties, developed and did not deviate for "his whole life through" from a sublimation served by the defenses of repression, displacement, and symbolization. He turned that which troubled him into an image or a poem; displaced, if need be, from the affect ridden form that threatened to trouble and emerge from his unconscious (memory). Freed thus from persistent memories invading from the prison of his past, Goethe could shape his reality, become busy with the world and free to roam. He often traveled. For instance, he left a lover without warning for a two year sojourn through Italy in is mid-thirties.

Goethe's attitude toward marriage is contained in this quote-

"Love is an ideal thing. Marriage is reality". Avoidance of marriage permeated his life and works. I have yet to find a literary work by Goethe in which the protagonists marry. In "Hermann and Dorothea"

Goethe (1797) Kindle loc. 10648]

preparation for marriage occurs. Emphasis is placed on the danger of loss of individuality for the potential spouse. Congreve (1700), who never married, expressed the problem in his well known phrase from "The Way of the World", "… before I may by degrees dwindle to a wife." 1

Goethe lived with Christine Volpius, whom he met in 1788, for 18 years before he married her at the request of their son. She died two years later.

The Transition To Mastery Through Art

The transition to mastery through art from neurotic expressions, which repeat fantasies through life altering behavior changes such as hypochondriasis, and self destructive behavior, can be seen in the novel "The Sorrows of Young Werther".

Date (1774)

Kindle Loc. 7620

Precis - Werther falls in love with Lotte in Weimar. She is engaged. He courts her. She rejects him. He commits suicide.

Life events - Goethe was in love with an engaged woman who rejected him. He was depressed. Instead of suicide, he conflated his experience with that of a lawyer friend named Jerusalem, who had become depressed after his rejection by a married woman, and had committed suicide. The book became a worldwide success. It was banned in Japan as a means of controlling suicide. Goethe mastered rejection by writing about suicide.

MEMORY BORNE THEMES THAT ARE EXPRESSED IN GOETHE'S WRITINGS

The unconscious affects and fantasy themes with childhood antecedents that can be found in Goethe's writings described below are:

A threatening power figure

The stolen child

The Murdered child

Darkness enhancing distortion

Loneliness and longing

WRITINGS

GOETHE IN ITALY - "Erotica Romana"

Date (1790)

KINDLE Loc 10396

Precis- This poem is rich in the erotic lore of Greek mythology as background for telling the story of a love affair that Goethe shared with a young woman of Rome.

Life events- In 1786 Goethe, aged 38, left Weimar for a two years (1786-1788) sojourn in Italy. He had had an ongoing relationship with Charlotte, the lady in waiting for Barones von Stein, who did not accompany him in Italy. They had met in 1776. The relationship ended in 1789. Mazzarello (2010) has written a study of the two year journey. He concluded that Goethe withdrew from relationships with women when he found that a potential lover had a fiancée or boyfriend, and that there was evidence that Goethe suffered from generalized anxiety.

There is another description of Goethe on that journey in which he is presented as a assertive and successful lover. Written by Goethe (1790), it is called "Erotica Romana" Kindle loc. 10396, 10558. It is primarily a poem dedicated to a current and undistorted erotic reality. One stanza catches our eye. It tells of an evening when his lover fails to appear. His distress at her behavior fades as he realizes that her guardian is there in her place; *a threatening power figure offering danger instead of love.*

Goethe, J. *"Faust, Part 1*

Date (1808)

Kindle Loc.5896

Precis- Faust is old. He longs for youth. The devil appears. He offers Faust youth and a beautiful girl as payment for Faust's soul. Faust accepts. He becomes young. He impregnates the girl. He leaves with the devil. The girl kills the baby. Faust and the devil come to the prison in which she is held. They try to free her. She refuses. She is welcomed into heaven. They depart before the coming of the dawn.

The story is traditional. Goethe added one element to the myth. This was the character of the girl, named Gretchen.

Butler (1948) in the "The Myth of the Magus" traces the Faust myth to its ancient beginnings. There was never a girl. The addition by Goethe of the child, who is murdered, is a mastery intrusion from childhood, when he experienced the vulnerability, of a child in darkness, to the dangers of threatening beings.

Goethe, J. Title "Ehrlenkoenig"

Date (1782)

Kindle Loc. 11566

Precis- A father carries his son on horseback swiftly through the dark windy night. The child is ill. They are riding to home. The boy tells his father that he hears the voice of the Ehrlenkoenig calling softly to him. The demon offers to take the child with him to a place where he can play with his daughters. The father tells the boy to be calm. As they come to their home, the boy dies.

Life events- Goethe had had a recent life threatening experience during the night in which he experienced a massive hemorrhage. Recovery took a year and a half. The Ehrlenkoenig was a well known Danish myth about a demon who stole children.

Mastery intrusions from childhood- In the darkness, the four year old child was frightened by a projection of hostility, that took the form of a demon, who we can see from his derived adult fantasies, invites a child to come with him, as did the Ehrlenkoenig.

Goethe, J. Title- "Wilhelm Meister, Years of Apprenticeship Vols.2-3.

Wilhelm Meister was written over many years. It was printed in six volumes. Mignon is a primary character. She represents a displaced mastery of Goethe's early life experiences.

Date (1829)

Kindle Loc. See Bibliography

Precis - Wilhelm Meister was a young man, who was sent on a voyage of apprenticeship to collect debts owed to his family. During the course of a year, he experiences, grows and matures. One day, while with a friend near a public square, he came upon a group of performing acrobats. Among them was a girl of twelve or thirteen years of age, whom he had seen perform. She was being beaten with the handle of a whip by one of the acrobats. Wilhelm stopped him violently. The child disappeared into the crowd. Asking the acrobat "where you stole her?" (Goethe (1828) Vol. one, page 92) Wilhelm bought her from her persecutor. Through two volumes, Mignon, for that was her name, flickered through many pages, serving Wilhelm, loving Wilhelm, seeking in him her lost father. Always sad and deserted, her loneliness and longing [sehnsucht] were expressed in songs that asked about the land from which she had been stolen. ["Do you know a place somewhere, where lemon trees are growing"] and expressed her longing. ["None but the lonely heart can know my sorrow."] Eventually she was placed, along with Wilhelm's natural son, Felix, in the home of a friend. Careful questions by the friend resulted in confirmation that Mignon had indeed been stolen at an early age from the Milan area by acrobats. Away from Wilhelm, she lost control, for the "… presence of a loved one can deprive the imagination of its destructive force and convert desire into quiet contemplation.", [Vol. Three page 90] She failed, dwindled, and withered. When confronted with a potential bride for Wilhelm, she collapsed and died.[page 105] Wilhelm went to the child saying, "Let me see the child that I have killed" [Vol three page 106.]

One character (Mignon) in "Wilhelm Meister" expressed the fears of being stolen or killed and the lonely longings that were encoded in memory in Goethe's early childhood.

Impact: Thomas, L (1866) adapted the story of Mignon for his opera "Mignon". In the opera Mignon is beautiful, nubile, flirtatious, and by the end of the opera, married to Wilhelm Meister.

Goethe, J. Title *"Faust, Part 2"*

Date (1833)

Kindle Loc. 5896

Precis - Free from the devil's presence, Faust seeks absolution through good works. One attempt draws our attention. He tried to make a baby to replace Grechen's murdered child. He created a homunculus. This was an act of artistic plastic creativity. It could not live. Books discharge an author's tensions. They do not bring babes back to life. Faust went on to seek further acts of absolution..

Life events - Faust was written over many years,

Mastery intrusions from childhood - Mastery of the fear that a child could be stolen or murdered took the form of '. creation of a homunculus to replace the murdered child.

Theory and Therapy

We have seen in Goethe's time many forms of therapy. Each is based on a then contemporary idea of that which mental illness was.

> Goethe and is father used behavior modification.

> Goethe used desensitizing.

> Goethe's mother used friendly bribery when she offered peaches.

> Voyages and focus on reality were recommended.

Decathexis of fantasy and mood through cathexes of current reality, future planning, group participation, and "Religious meditation.

Joining a group that directed attention to others through criticizing them. (Goethe KINDLE Loc. 532) "In my efforts to free myself from the pressure of the too gloomy and powerful, which continued to rule within me, and seemed to me sometimes as strength, sometimes as weakness, I was thoroughly assisted by that open, social, stirring manner of life, which attracted me more and more, to which I accustomed myself, and which I at last learned to enjoy with perfect freedom. It is not difficult to remark in the world, that man feels himself most freely and most perfectly rid of his own feelings when he represents to himself the faults of others, and expatiates upon them with complacent censoriousness. "It is a tolerably pleasant sensation even to set ourselves above our equals by disapprobation and misrepresentation; for which reason good society, whether it consists of few or many, is most delighted with it. But nothing equals the comfortable self-complacency, when we erect ourselves into judges of our superiors, and of those who are set over us,--of princes and statesmen, --when we find public institutions unfit and injudicious, only consider the possible and actual obstacles, and recognize neither the greatness of the invention, nor the co-operation which is to be expected from time and circumstances in every undertaking."

Another emphasis away from neurotic pressures in the eighteenth century was participation in religious belief. Formal religious belief offered "a place of habitation, and a name" for spiritual feelings and offered a theory of causation for mental illness. As an orientation in dealing with fears and uncomfortable affects, religion offers a theory to support exorcism and meditation. Goethe described such a meditation.

GOETHE KINDLE Loc. 5266.

"One easily sees how the redemption is not only decreed from eternity, but is considered as eternally necessary,--nay, that it must ever renew itself through the whole time of generation and existence. In this view of the subject, nothing is more natural than for the Divinity himself to take the form of man, which had already prepared itself as a veil, and to share his fate for a short time, in order, by this assimilation, to enhance his joys and alleviate his sorrows. The history of all religions and philosophies teaches us, that this great truth, indispensable to man, has been handed down by different nations, in different times, in various ways, and even in strange fables and images, in accordance with their limited knowledge: enough, if it only be acknowledged that we find ourselves in a condition which, even if it seems to drag us down and oppress us, yet gives us opportunity, nay, even makes it our duty, to raise ourselves up, and to fulfill the purposes of the Godhead in this manner, that, while we are compelled on the one hand to concentrate ourselves (/uns zu verselbsten/), we, on the other hand, do not omit to expand ourselves (/uns zu entselbstigen/) in regular pulsation"

CONCLUSION

Before dynamic theory was discovered by Freud, Childhood Psychopathology was seen to be a product of willfulness, religious demon intrusion, laziness, and social misdirection. The therapies of the time were derived from the theories of the time. Unconscious motivation existed, but was not recognized by science as a factor contributing to psychopathology. Goethe (1811-1830 kindle Loc 12) described neurotic signs and symptoms at different stages of his life. Current diagnostic entities were present. The life situations and stresses relating to the time of the onset of pathology could be identified. Their encoding in memory (the unconscious) could be detected through exploration of their return to consciousness in displaced form in psychopathology and sublimative creativity such as poems, plays, and novels. When insight into unconscious motivation as a generator of psychopathology became an orientation, exploration and amelioration of unconscious factors, through dynamic child therapy, was added to the child psychotherapy armamentarium.

JDS Is the idea of child development so new? When was the idea first introduced? What were the theories that informed perception and caused knowledge of childhood to be diverted?

CAS As far as I have been able to understand it, developmental child growth, as a concept, has existed only since the early nineteen hundreds. It begins with the psychoanalytic observation that remnants of the developmental growth of early childhood influence adult mental life. Prior to this beginning and persisting for most of the world's religions to this day is the theory that organisms develop from homunculi, that have existed since the beginning of creation. Scholars call this belief "preformism"; an academic ghost town, which is rarely visited. In common belief, preformism, is an influential world pervasive concept. Evidence of its presence, both in the past and present,. can be detected from a study of its derivatives:

In the "Malleus Maleficarum", a 1487 guide to the identification of witches that sat on the desk of every judge in Christendum, the question is raised, Can a child be conceived through intercourse with an incubus? Such a child would be called a "cambion".

The influences of such a union on the characteristics of the child were thought to bypass developmental influences. For instance, a woman (Vivian), whom he loved, rejected Merlin, a cambion, because of the evil to be expected from such a person.

Leeuwenhoek, the Dutch 1677 microscopist, reported that he had seen in sperm cells tiny creatures with adult forms ready to grow in size from birth on.

Reflections of the belief that the child is fully formed at birth and can grow quickly to full size can be found in fairy tales, such as the Chinese story of "Neszha Stirs Up the Sea", and the Russion tale "Tsar Saltan" of Pushkin.

Tagore, the Hindu poet wrote the poem "The Beginning" collected in the book, "The Crescent Moon". In the poem a child asks his mother "Where have I come from…..?". The mother responds "You were in the dolls of my childhood games…" reflecting the concept of preexistence. The title of the book is of interest to us. The crescent moon is the Hindu symbol for childhood. Siva, the god of childhood, wears a crescent moon in his hair (Siva Naturaj)

Freud at first favored Lamarkian "inheritance of acquired characteristics." Evidence of the persistence of this theory can be found in "Moses and Monotheism".

The Darwinian concept of an adaptational evolution of the form of species, introduced a challenge to the concept of the preformed human in 1870.. The finding of gills in embryos, which developed into branchial clefts, was another challenging factor. For early psychoanalysts, the door was open to a reorganization of knowledge of human behavior that placed emphasis on developmental influences during years of growth on character, behavior, and mental illness.

BIOGRAPHICAL REFERENCE TO CHILDHOOD FANTASY RESOLUTION

Biographies of writers describe the role of waking latency age fantasy in the day to day resolution of trauma in children; outside the clinical setting. Kinkaid (1991) in reviewing a biography of Trollope by Hall(1991) describes Trollope as having a childhood where "...humiliation loaded on the child through all his school years; the beatings and desolation; the turn of the heartsick and friendless little boy to an inward life of tale-spinning, where he could do clever things and win approval - where "beautiful young women used to be fond of me." (Kinkaid (P16)/ (Hall (P30). As an adult, Trollope wrote 47 novels which contain reflections of his childhood's pain.

Hoffman (1991) in reviewing a biography of Poe by Silverman (1991) tells us that: "...Poe's mother died when he was three years old. -he never resolved his bereavement." (P 17). Silverman (1991) describes the role of childhood trauma in determining adult psychopathology in what follows: "Much of Edgar's career, too might be understood as a sort of prolonged mourning, an artistic brooding - on an assemblage of fantasies activated by an ever - living past. As no product of his imagination would put to right what had gone wrong or restore what he had once possessed, he would begin over and over, repeating in new forms, different imagery, and fresh characters and scenes of dilemma which he presented as the peculiar condition of his existence." (page 78)

APPENDICES

APPENDIX ONE

"THE ORIGINS OF CERTAINTY"

ooooooooo

This Appendix is an edited version of a paper presented to the INTERNATIONAL PSYCHOANALYTIC ASSOCIATION 2015 BOSTON meeting.

> "The eye sees only what the mind is prepared to comprehend".

> Robertson Davies

"THE ORIGINS OF CERTAINTY"

Fixation and regression to developmental levels of psychosexual development shape emotional and fantasy responses in later life. In like manner, fixation and regression to the stages of memory encoding and object relations in the early years of life, provide a paradigm for informed memory and its interpretation of new experiences throughout life.

PRIMARY CERTAINTY ESTABLISHING CERTAINTY IN CHILDHOOD

At first breath, the human infant is limited to encoding into (haptic) memory, internally experienced sensations, which when recalled are sensed to be as real as pain. Why? Because they are real. This is called physiological memory. By one and a half years, a few muffled words acquired through telereceptor sensory inputs (sight and sound) begin to be encoded in an amalgam of affects and images acquired through sight or sound. Both elements of the amalgam share and convey physiological memory's sense of reality.

Physiological memory components feel real because they represent internal reality. This internal physiological feeling, when blended with word content, introduces a sense of certainty to the remembered word and the concept it represents.

By approximately 23 months of age, encoding in memory is achieved through recognizable words; blended with physiological sensations. This combination is a transitional form of remembering. It exists during the shift from physiological encoding of haptic based memory sensations to the full ability to think and to speak in words without affects, as is found in abstract thinking.

Blending, of a physiological component with a word representation, results in a memory entity that is experienced as certain. The participation in blended memory moieties (words and affects) of previously experienced internal sensations,

transfers a narcissistic sense of certainty to the
word contents representing memory.

Certainty is derived from the intuitive conclusion
that repeatability verifies. The most important
memory contents acquired are precipitates of
repeated experiences and the often repeated comments
of parents from which world view, identity, and
self image are forged. The most important of the
precipitates are the political self, the sexual
self, and the self as a part of a nation or subject
of a king for whom one would die. Both recalled
and activated memories encoded during this period
of transition are believed with certainty to be
unchallengeable. Whether they are fixated memories
or the products of regression, these memories are
experienced as real, immutable, and not subject to
rational investigation. This is why it is commonly
said, "Do not argue about politics or religion".

Memories are linked to certainty, when physiological
sensations (affects) are blended with word phrases
and concepts. Certainty affects are shared, when
both components enter awareness simultaneously.
This experience of certainty without proof is a
paradigm for the establishment of certainty, when
in later times in life, the child faces situations
which are potentially linked with doubt. It offers
a way to replace doubt with certainty. This can
support a life long state of identity from which
to launch secure forays into the real world. Self
images derived from one's identity exert a powerful
pull on determining the direction taken by cathexes
in selecting objects and in planning.. They dominate

a person's theories about new perceptions and are the generator of self fulfilling prophesies. They drive internally generated fate. Such certainty experience is called **primary certainty.**

SECONDARY CERTAINTY

ESTABLISHIG CERTAINTY IN ADULTHOOD

If there is no objective information to use in later life for the establishment of reality about declarations of love, religious truths such as the existence and actions of god, proof of paternity, and conclusions drawn from testimony in a court of law, certainty can be secondarily achieved through the use of tokens and oaths. The longer ago and the less science available, the more are tokens of proof required for the establishment of certainty. Since the ability to believe, defend, and even die for or kill for a false belief is a universal human trait, it is important to identify and to understand the tokens that "verify" false beliefs and their role in superstition, mythology, war, sexuality, political identity, religion, and parenthood. False certainty strengthened by tokens threatens potentially disruptive intrusions into the Psychoanalytic process. (See example 2 below)

Determining truth through tokens, which "verify certainty", long preceded reality testing; as a determinant of truth for mankind. Reality testing first appears in the works of Aristotle in @300 BC. Developmental characteristics of the sense of reality were first discussed by Ferenczi (1913).

IDENTITY CERTAINTY

EXAMPLE ONE - (CULTURAL)

Tribal man lived a hunting life guided by superstition, which explained origins and culturally important rituals needed for survival. The overall life and identity of each person was dominated by the certainty of their governing myths. Individuals survived in personal encounters with the dangers of the hunt by a personalized approach to the reality of immediate dangers that could be seen and heard.

Emerging from a twenty day sojourn through the jungles of the Okavanga Delta in Botswana, Africa, I found myself at the hut of a San tribesman deep in the Kalahari desert. During a prearranged visit, he showed me how to find trap-door spider nests, how to build traps for birds out of the flexible reeds of a desert oasis, and he cut into plants to produce water. Through my time in the jungle all that I needed had been flown in. In the desert, this man, carrying nothing but a sharpened digging stick, commanded the reality of the desert and survived.

As we parted, the impact on his life of primary certainty appeared. He asked me in a begging tone to tell the people of America of his plight. Said he, "They have moved my family from our home. They have moved us to a concrete building in a distant valley. How can we live? I don't know which tree to avoid, or which rock to pray to, when I want to hunt." Belief, remembered with certainty, took priority in his thinking.

Superstitious beliefs dominated the intuitive perception of reality in the ancient world. This set the stage for Plato's **[Phaedrus (Ant)]** dictum that endowed knowledge taught by elders was the only truth. This world view was challenged by Aristotle (300 BC), who in stripping away the prescriptive sanctities of endowed myth, sought reality in the world of remembered experience. He denied syllogism and accepted only that which was verifiable, repeatable, and transmissible. Unfortunately events did not support him. Epidemics were blamed on gods (mythic figures). When he died, scientific truth died with him. St. Augustine (400 AD), seven hundred years later proclaimed that the only truth was the Bible. Disbelief was heresy; punishable by death. Four hundred years later St. Thomas Aquinas (1256-9) reopened the door for Aristotelian science to join myth as a tolerated element in two sharply contradictory dual sourced realities.

PRIMARY CERTAINTY SUPPORTS DUAL REALITY

Western Civilization is characterized by the presence of a dual system for arriving at a sense of reality.

In the first system, there is an infused reality, passed down by parents, teachers and keepers of faith, through mythological conventions. These teachings become the basis for a mythically determined part of a culturally shared "mother landscape" (Spengler 1922) for use in evaluating the "reality" of new information and for creating compatible explanations for eldritch natural phenomena, such as Niobe's despair as the source of weeping stones.

In the second system, explorations of the world matrix have been codified to create the part of the "mother landscape" that is the shared scientific world view, against which the reality value of new interpretations of inputs can be judged.

This state of affairs has provided the supportive philosophical basis for the current stage of Western Civilization, in which the certainty of religious beliefs, and superstitions, exist side by side with scientific proofs and theories.

EXAMPLE TWO — (CLINICAL)

Dual Reality As a Problem In Child Therapy

During a discussion about lateness with an eight year old patient, there was introduced the topic of the great glacier, which had left the hill on which my office stood and which had delayed his arrival that day. I explained that the glacier had been at its height ten thousand years ago and had left this hill (a terminal moraine) as it receded. He mused half to himself. "5750 years" was what I think I heard. He repeatedly mumbled the number. He clearly was bewildered. Finally he spoke up, explaining to me that I must be wrong for God created the earth some 5700 years ago and "There was no earth ten thousand years ago". His referent for reality and mine differed. His sense of reality used transcendent concepts as the basis for comparison in the evaluation of the reality of new inputs. My manifest verbal symbolic forms used the conventions of "scientific objective natural reality" as the basis for comparison in the evaluation of the reality of new inputs. If the gauntlet dropped by the boy had been picked up, it would have undermined the therapy.

An amalgam of maturation and tradition shapes the content, form, and boundaries of ontogenetic development. Psychotherapy as a scientific discipline intrudes on the products of this process. At times this creates a stress for the therapist-parent-patient bond. Persistence of the primary certainty of early stage memory influences beliefs, fantasies, and interpretation of new experiences. The illusion of reality is supported by certainty. Certainty linked to encoded memory, when recalled as a mechanism to support fantasy and expectations, creates an impenetrable boundary in the way of attempts to replace false hope with reality. The parent-society-child bond that supports resolution of doubt with false hope is intruded upon at the therapist's peril.

Normal maturation takes a child from the haptic experienced self and fantasy to externally directed cathexes which give priority to the telereceptor channels that deliver external reality to awareness. The transition from living in one's fantasies to living in the world entails valuing consistency over probability. Arrival at the autonomy of thought that occurs when every concrescence of myth is stripped away is an essential part of "The emancipation of thought from myth," [Frankfort (1977 p 386)] Persistence of the tendency to assign certainty to fantasy and superstition in the face of data that can be experienced, repeated, transmitted, and communicated undermines the path to maturity. Psychodynamic Psychotherapy aims at reversing this process. Aristotle's critique of mythic thinking, "A single sparrow does not make a spring." is applicable here.

A conflict can appear while conducting treatment. The encouragement of reality testing can undermine family ties. Attempts by a therapist to challenge ideation that glues the family together and makes it part of a social network, such as religious or political belief, may result in the withdrawal of the child from treatment by the parent. The creation of identity from these beliefs is part of age appropriate behavior. Teaching clergy are quoted as saying "Give me the child before he is five and I'll have him for life." Societies introduce children to local ideology that is imbued with the feeling that they are certain and irreplaceable. They create local group beliefs that being certain support institutions, love, buildings, forgiveness, group loyalty, combat, murder and war. They provide beliefs to live or die by. Challenge of such group beliefs entails the possibility of undermining socialization in the child patient. Reality, on the other hand provides knowledge to share that can, when held in common, support universally agreed upon and held concepts. This could encourage peaceful sharing.

SECONDARY CERTAINTY

The possibility of activation of certainty in adulthood is a remnant of early childhood certainty. Then, certainty associated with a belief without proof, was the product of the persistence of haptic (internal) feelings. Such feelings persisted, when linked to words, when words were added to memory. A persistent remnant of this process became a paradigm for use in creating certainty in resolving doubts encountered, when dealing with teaching beliefs, which stray from the data of scientific reality. To strengthen the quality of felt reality in later years, a token or an oath is employed to reinforce certainty to the level of that which was experienced during primary certainty.

SECONDARY CERTAINTY IN HISTORY AND LITERATURE

Where there is doubt about religious belief, paternity, legal opinion, political ideas, and declarations of fated love, in times before science could provide clarifications, rituals or tokens were used to support certainty. Examples In history and literature of this way of resolving uncertainty and doubt are presented below.

TOKENS SUPPORT CERTAINTY FOR RELIGIOUS BELIEF

(7ᵀᴴ CENTURY BC REPORTING ON THE EVENTS OF 1300BC)

God's promise to be with Moses was made a certainty when God said,

"*Certainly* I will be with thee; and this shall be a *token* unto thee, that I have sent thee: When thou hast brought forth the people out of Egypt, ye shall serve God upon this mountain. [Exodus3:12]

ESTABISHING CERTAINTY OF FATHERHOOD

Before there was a scientific means for establishing fatherhood, tokens were used to reinforce certainty about the identity of the father.

In The "Old Testament" this is portrayed in The Story of Tamar, {the widow of Onan.} Tamar, was held back from marrying by her father-in law. She dressed as a prostitute and sat by a path that she knew he would take. He did not recognize her. He went in unto her. She demanded a kid (baby goat) in payment. Having no kid, he promised payment the next day, leaving tokens as testimony to his good intent. His agents could not find her the next day. She returned home. Soon pregnancy showed. Her father-in-law condemned her to death. She showed him his tokens. Abashed, he withdrew his verdict.

In the Mahabharata this use of tokens is portrayed in the story of Sakuntali {the mother of Bharata) She was the daughter of a Hindu holy man. A passing prince convinced her that they were married, leaving tokens to provide certainty of marriage. He impregnated her. When a baby was born, she visited the prince. He denied fatherhood. She showed him his tokens. He accepted the child as his own.

CERTAINTY IN THE CONCLUSIONS DERIVED FROM TESTIMONY

UNDER OATH -

This is portrayed in the story of "SUSANNA AND THE ELDERS", In the Old Testament Apocrypha

The story of "Susanna and the Elders" tells of a young married woman living in Babylon during the first exile of the Jewish people (The Babylonian captivity after 586 BCE.). - Susanna was in her garden. She sent her maids into the house to fetch oil and perfumes for her bath. Two lecherous elders spied on her. They planned to force her to submit to them sexually. They threaten that, if she refused, they would denounce her as an adulteress, Adultery was, in ancient Jewish law, a capital crime for women. The elders threatened that they would name a partner whom they would say was with her under a tree. Susanna refused, preferring death over sin. She was falsely accused by the elders and condemned to death. The judge Daniel, vindicated Susanna. He exposed the elders' mendacity by interrogating them under oath separately. When he asked "Under which tree did you see Susanna in sin?", each named a different kind of tree. Susanna's virtue was made certain. As false witnesses, the elders were executed.

A GRANDIOSE TOKEN SUPPORTING CERTAINTY IN VALIDATING LOVE

In Rupert Brook's POEM "THE CALL"

"Out of the nothingness of sleep,
The slow dreams of Eternity,
There was a thunder on the deep:
I came, because you called to me.
I broke the Night's primeval bars,
I dared the old abysmal curse,
And flashed through ranks of frightened stars
Suddenly on the universe!

The eternal silences were broken;
Hell became Heaven as I passed.
What shall I give you as a *token*,
A *sign* that we have met, at last?

I'll write upon the shrinking skies
The scarlet splendour of your name."

OTHER PHENOMENA WITH ROOTS IN EARLY TRANSITIONAL BLENDING OF PHYSIOLOGICAL AND VERBAL MEMORY

PARANOID CERTAINTY

Certainty turns the assertive products of projection into paranoid accusations. Projection begins when the first intermediate phase of the transition that adds words to sensations in memory occurs. Then the experience of thought changes.

A boundary, differentiating inside (Haptic) from outside (telereceptor) develops. Projection of physiologically based instinctual pressure, aggressive or sexual, across this boundary between the self and the object world becomes possible. Across this boundary inner feelings can be experienced as belonging to a world beyond the self. The boundary is established when the child can experience telereceptor [external] sensations from the outside as differenciated from haptic [internal] sensations on the inside.

Hearing and vision provide the child with evidence of a newly identified zone beyond the boundary of the self, across which drives and concepts (haptic content) can be projected. A physiological reality feeling component, present on the haptic side of the boundary can accompany the projected haptic content. Physiological reality feelings of certainty can be generalized beyond the ego boundary to color words and ideas in consciousness till they are certainty-affect laden.

Reality testing is immature, when feelings of certainty associated with physiological memory can be generalized to new ideas and words. The process of linking words, motives, and ideas in awareness, to certainty of its reality is the process by which projected elements are converted to paranoid constructs. Certainty-affect reinforces the impact of the word component of projected content.

The introduction of verbal memory reinforces ego boundaries. The blending of internal sensations with words, during encoding and recall of memories, imparts the reality of haptic sensing to associated words. Why, one might ask, does this not happen earlier?. Feelings [anger for instance] are haptic. Words enter the zone of awareness through sight and sound (telereceptor) input, This occurs at about 2 years of age.. This particular ego boundary cannot exist before the zone of words comes into being.

Projection reinforced by primary certainty is age appropriate when fantasy formation is accepted as a mechanism that helps adjustment. Immature [latency] children deal with frustration presented by inaccessible reality through fantasy. In adolescence projection into believed fantasy becomes pathological, when it distracts (counter-cathexis) from and increasingly interferes with the expression of drives in reality.

PSYCHOSOMATIC SYMPTOMS.

Regression to early memory organizations enables primitive thinking. One such memory organization characterizes thinking at the time that words are activated to blend with somatic sensations in the expression of encoded memory. Either somatic expression ["manifest signs"] or words ["manifest symptoms"] can express drives, fantasies, and recalls. Shifts within the blend of word expression and somatic expression occur in response to fear of the aggression or sexuality or world destruction connected to the words of a fantasy. A shift from verbal expression to somatization suppresses awareness of feared uncomfortable affects. This permits the achievement of expression of drive derivatives hidden from awareness and protects objects in reality.

An example of this process follows. A nineteen year old patient interrupted her associations to experienced abortions with the command "look". She simultaneously pointed to a giant hive that was rising on her forearm. I asked her **What were you thinking just before this happened?"** Answered she, "I was thinking – 'I'd like to rip your guts out like they did mine" As she said this return to expression through words, the hive receded. Notice that my comment asked her to reverse her shift from verbal expression to somatization, which had defensively suppressed awareness of uncomfortable affects.

CONSCIOUSNESS

Clinical "consciousness" varies in content and in the mechanisms that alter awareness according to each stage of life achieved. There are four stages of experienced consciousness that accompany the addition of verbal (telerecptor) components to encoding and recall.

These are –

One – In the preverbal stage internal (haptic) physiological sensation encodes experience. Perception and response can be detected as evidence of consciousness. An example is the feeling of hunger which activates crying. Few words such as mama and milk are present. They are used for immediate demands. They do not participate in future planning.

Two - At about 23 months verbal representation is blended into the process of encoding. Certainty is attributed to words as a result of blending. Memory content can be transmitted verbally to others. Verbalization makes shared awareness reportable. This provides reportable evidence of consciousness. An example is requests to know the names of things pointed to. Words are used to express immediate demands. They do not participate in future planning. Shifts between verbal and physiological expression of ideas and urges in fantasy occur continuously.

Three- The addition of words to the processes of encoding and remembering introduces the idea of two spatial sources for perceptions; inside and outside the self. From inside comes physiological sensation felt as certain and linked words which have been encoded in memory. The latter may be neutral; exemplified by numbers and rote learning that can enter awareness without censorship or they may be linked to physiological sensation, such as certainty and anxiety. From outside comes new experience and new words. Words from outside introduce an inside and outside to awareness, resulting in the creation of an ego boundary across which internal content can be projected. Associated certainty feelings turn projection into paranoia.

Four- Conscious awareness is total during the early years of encoding and remembering, when it is not truncated by symbolization. The latter does not become active until at 26 months (see Sarnoff

1970B). It is also not truncated by repression, which becomes active at 4 years (Piaget 1945) Awareness truncated by symbolism and repression, denial, and suppression, which is strained through perception informed by memory, is adult consciousness.

SUMMARY AND CONCLUSIONS00

Early in the third year of life, the encoding in memory of events experienced and descriptions of self overheard, changes. Encoding through word meanings is blended with physical sensation encoding. The existing physiological component contributes a narcissistic sense of certainty to the blend. Attitudes toward identity, sexuality, religious belief, and political identity forged during this period can persist throughout life as part of one's identity. This is called primary certainty. Memory content accompanied by this sense of certainty is experienced in later years as beyond challenge, immutable and not subject to rational logic. When faced with adult situations seeped with the possibility of doubt, such as fatherhood, declarations of love, religious dogma, conclusions from courtroom testimony, and national identity, tokens and oaths can be used to recreate the certainty experience of early childhood. This is called secondary certainty.

APPENDIX TWO

CHARTS

Human awareness is first drawn to physical
sensations such as hunger, loneliness, and muscle
tone. These are actual sensations. Since sensation
is incontrovertible, they are experienced as real.
These sensations are encoded in memory for use
in recognition of sensations and new experiences.
By the second year of life, a maturational factor
enhances the encoding of experience into memory.
That factor is the word. Words, locked to explanatory
meanings, provided by caretakers, are imbedded in
memory with physical feelings. These word linked
meanings reflect attitudes characteristic of the
caretakers. They often contain strongly held beliefs.
Explanations in verbal form, based on social
mythological beliefs, become linked syncretically
with feelings in encoded memory. Linking of feelings
to concepts, experienced in words, creates a new
entity. This entity expresses in one unit the shared
characteristics of its two sources. One of these
carried-over characteristics is a sense of reality,
which comes to be shared. The individuality of the
person surrenders to form, as linked feeling/verbal
memory are saddled with a feeling of reality. In the

words of Stefan Zweig (1976), It is then that "The grain of dust that was man [is] no longer counted today as a creature of volition."

When verbal explanations and attitudes (political beliefs, religious dogma, patrimony, nationality) are recalled later throughout life, the linked feeling of a sense that "This is real." arises to consciousness with them.

Word bound explanations from authorities that are linked to sensation take on this characteristic sensation. They are felt to be real. Whether they remain in consciousness as the result of fixation or return to consciousness as the result of regression organized mythological structure retained in later years, the reality of myths of identity (religious, political, patrimony, nationality) can be strong enough to support anger, war, and murder such as burning at the stake.

Feelings of wonder and of reality surrender their individual power to attract awareness, when explanation or experience is vented through fantasy play (abreaction) or is confronted with shared insights expressed in words. Shared concepts during child therapy introduce a newly shared level of the sense of reality. This diminishes doubt about arbitrary and irrational beliefs, which had been controlled through arbitrary rituals and beliefs. Energy is freed to deal with the world and reality, New remembered word explanations replace sound bites and ritual.

With cognitive maturity concrete recall of word elements in memory gives way to memory of abstract concepts. Eventually reality replaces endowment. Then true reality testing based on actual reality (physis) is achieved, and object choices free of fantasy influences become possible. Regression along this developmental line supports mob psychology. The transition, in parallel, of the decline of the sense of reality and its replacement by reality testing is traced in the following charts.

CHART ONE

///

ZONE	AGE	VERBAL SKILL LEVEL	ENCODING	CATHEXIS	PSYCHO-SEXUAL LEVEL

///

PRENATAL THROUGH PREVEBAL

ZONE	AGE	VERBAL SKILL LEVEL	ENCODING	CATHEXIS	PSYCHO-SEXUAL LEVEL
A	-minus 3mos to 2 yrs 6mos	Pre-natal to Peri-Early Verbal	Physical to Physio-Verbal	Self Directed Soma Speaks Passive	Oral Syncretic,
					Emunctory Functions and Feeding Dependence

///

VERBAL ENCODING BEGOINS
"EMOTIONAL BECOMES RATIONAL"
THROUGH SHARED VERBALIZATION
MEMORY PERSISTENCE THROUGH FIXATION BEGINS

B	2yrs 6 mos	Words and	Physical and	Centered on	Anal
	to 4 yrs	Mumbling	Words	Supporting	Self Controlled
		to Clear Words &		Objects	Emunctory
		Simple Symbols	Which	Introduce	Functions
			Endowed Beliefs which are Retained as Real		Achieved Control Self-Object Differentiation

———————————————————————————————————————

///

WEAK REPRESSION

C	4 yrs	Cryptic	Dream Words,	Endowed Beliefs &	Phallic
	To 6 yrs.	Symbols	Sound	Self Evolved	Competition
			Bites	Fantasies	Two Person Fantasies

———————————————————————————————————————

///

STRONG REPRESSION
RECOVERY thru "REGRESSION
TO FANTASY" {Latency}

D	6 yrs to 8 yrs	Latency Fantasy as Defense	Myths & Endowed Knowledge. End of Consciousness Expansion with Diminished Recall (Repression) Visual and Verbal Memory.	Pre-informed Interpretation of new Experiences	Oedipal Competition Three Person Fantasies

//

INCREASED INFLUENCE OF REALITY
ON CHOICE OF FANTASY SYMBOLS
{LATE LATENCY}

E	8 yrs to 11 yrs	Humanoid Persecutors Future Perceptions and Identity -Memory Panels-	Shared Endowed Beliefs, Sensed as Real, are Used for Interpretation of	Interpretation of New Inputs Shared Concepts

//

ADOLESCENT INSTINCT REINFORCEMENT
INTENSIFIES SEEKING OBJECTS IN REALITY

F	11 YRS	Words as	Mixture of	Crushes
	To 15 yrs	Symbols of	Object Reality	Guided Interpretatin
		Repressed Elements And as Realiity	with Preconceptions Modifies Encoded Representations As Well	Search Terms

1

//

MATURE
REALITY TESTING

				Career Choice	Sexual
G	15 YRS	Mature Object	Shared Reality	Mate Selection	Mature
	To 30 YRS	Seeking in	Based on	Insurance	Object
		Reality Transmssability	Reality	Seeking	
		Teamwork	Repeatability		in Reality
			& Verifiability.		Team Work
			Reality Supports Rationality		

//

CHART TWO

///

ZONE	AGE	DEGREE OF REALITY TESTING	CONCRETE /ABSTRACT CONTINUUM	PATHOLOGY FIXATION * REGRESSIVE

///

PRENATAL THROUGH PREVERBAL

A -3mos SOMATIC ENCODING

to 2yrs 6 mos

Narcissistic Non-verbal

Psychosomatic
with Poor Adjustment
*Psychosomatic
 with Intermittent
 Adjustment
Autistic Mute
*Malignant
 Depression
*Elective
 Mutism
*PTSD
Somatic Hallucinations
ADHD Type One
organic innate

///

VERBAL ENCODING BEGINS

2yrs 6 mos   "EMOTIONAL BECOMES RATIONAL"
To 4 yrs   THROUGH SHARED VERBALIZATION

PERSISTENCE THROUGH FIXATION BEGINS

B

Shared Reality In	Concrete	Autistic Verbal
Symbolic Forms,	Verbal	Asperger
Endowed Word		Pytophobia
Meanings, Shared		Displacement to Somatic
With Caretakers,		and Verbal Entities,
Create an		Projection to Objects
Idiosyncratic World		of Drive Feelings and
Image {MARA}		Recalled Entities,
Supported by		Feared Phobic Symbols
a Sense of Reality,		Religious Explanations
Which Cannot Be		Are Felt To Be
Denied		Incontrovertible
		And Become the
		Source of Identity,
		*Hallucinations
		*Delusions
		ADHD type two
		Parents overstimulate
		Child with nudity
		excitement brutality

///

WEAK REPRESSION

C 4 Yrs	Certainty is Linked	Pseudoabstract	Infantile Zoophobias
To 6 Yrs	to the Sense of	Concrete	Night Fears
	Reality		Projection Of Intents

Projection Of Intents
 *Paranoia
Religious Beliefs
And Borders
Support Murder,
And Condemnation
To Hell.
Childhood Schizophrenia
 *War
 *Persecution
  ADHD TYPE THREE-

a.. Child's capacity to
absorb pressure or to
escape into
symbolization and
fantasy has been
over-ridden by the
strength of
seduction.

                OR

There is
b. Lack of symbol
formation – leaving
aggressive poorly
displaced antisocial
fantasies and
reactions to be
acted out without
delay.

_____

///

STRONG REPRESSION

RECOVERY THRU "REGRESSION

TO FANTASY" (LATENCY)

LATENCY FANTASY AS DEFENCE

D

6 Yrs To 8 Yrs	Certainty Makes Fear Fantasies Feel Real World Image Continues	Abstract Numbers Strong Concrete Facts Pseudoabstract Identity Through Predicate Surface Characteristics	Cultural Identity Latency states

---

///

INCREASED INFLUENCE OF REALITY

IN THE CHOICE OF FANTASY SYMBOLS

(LATE LATENCY)

E 8 Yrs

to 11 Yrs

Thenceforth Endowed World Image Content, Meanings, and Explanations (Political, Religious, and Identity Based) Acquired in Zone B, When Suggested or Remembered, Counter Reality Influences, .. Maintain the Status Quo, And Establish Borders.	Identity Through Innate Characteristics. Begins True Abstraction	Reality Enhanced Planning

---

///

ADOLESCENT INSTINCT REINFORCEMENT
INTENSIFIES SEEKING OBJECTS IN REALITY

F 11Yrs To 15 Yrs	Shift of love Object from Fantasy Image Toward Real People	Proverb Interpretation is Consistently Possible

///

MATURITY
REALITY TESTING

		-
G 15 yrs To 30Yrs	Team Play, Object Love Attainable Career Goals	Couplehood, Marriage Life Insurance Fear of Flying Ementia Praecox

///

CHART THREE

///

ZONE	AGE SKILL LEVEL	VERBAL SUSTITUTE OBJECTS	INTERMEDIATE SYMBOL TYPES	LUDIC

///

PRENATAL THROUGH PREVEBAL

A -minus 3mos	Pre-natal to	syncretism no	
to 2 yrs 6mos	Peri-Early	border - touching hair	play objects
	Verbal	while nursing to	rings and bells
	Functions	rubbing blanket edge	without meanings
		representation	
		Toy animals with names	

///

VERBAL ENCODING BEGINS
"EMOTIONAL BECOMES RATIONAL"
THROUGH SHARED VERBALIZATION
MEMORY PERSISTENCE THROUGH FIXATION BEGINS

B 2yrs 6 mos	Words and	Blankets and	Symbols that represent
to 4 yrs	Mumbling	Toy animals that are carried,	object's motivations with transparent
		fed, and taught,	latent meanings
		and sometimes feared	available as answers to questions
		.. when they become non-self	and to be used for mastery through
		entities	fantasy -abreaction

///

WEAK REPRESSION

C 4 yrs Cryptic Dream
  To   Symbols
  6 yrs. Haptic Content based on memory.
         Interpreted through dream expansion
         using drawings
         Ludic symbols   Animal
         Content can also be influenced by persecutors
         Telereceptor influences.   Shadowy
                                    beings
                                    Latent content is
                                    hard to reach
                                    through questions.
                                    Cathartic mastery
                                    Through play
                                    (abreaction)
                                    is indicated.

_____

///

STRONGE REPRESSION
RECOVERY thru "REGRESSION
TO FANTASY" {Latency}

D 6 yrs   Latency Fantasy   Memory as Object Amorphous
  to 8 yrs as Defense   Objects equated through
                             persecutors

concrete use of predicates.

                             Discharge through
                             "Ludic symbol"
                             (abreaction based)
                             Play is the primary
                             Defense in facing
                             the adult populated
                             world.

_____

///

INCREASED INFLUENCE OF REALITY
ON CHOICE OF FANTASY SYMBOLS
{LATE LATENCY}

E 8 to 11 yrs	Humanoid Persecutors	Memory as object Objects equated through intrinsic characteristics Humanoid persecutors	Disharge and mastery through ludic fantasy is eroded by abstract constructions that identify themes

---

///

ADOLESCENT INSTINCT REINFORCEMENT
INTENSIFIES SEEKING OBJECTS IN REALITY

F 11 YRS To 15 yrs	Words as Symbols Repressed Elements And as Realiity Representations as well	Abstraction mature. The child leaves the playroom Motivations are identified. Objects are chosen with self gratification in mind.	Ludic Demise

---

///

MATURE
REALITY TESTING

G	15 YRS	Mature Object	Teamwork – the search for an object in terms of shared needs	Fantasy is lived out with new real people
	To 30 YRS	Seeking in Reality		

///

UNIT NINE -

BIBLIOGRAPHY

This Bibliography consists of two components. These are;

1. References related to the contents of this book.

2. Basic references related to the required knowledge needed for the practice of child psychotherapy.

BIBLIOGRAPHY

Abraham, K. (1924). A short study of the development of the libido in the light of mental disorders. Selected Papers of Karl Abraham. New York: Basic, 1954.

Anthony, E. J. (1959). An experimental approach to the psychopathology of childhood: sleep disturbances. British Journal of Medical Psychology 321: 19-37.

Bender, L (1947). Childhood Schizophrenia. Journal of the Academy of Orthopsychiatry 17: 40-56.

Bender, L. (1970). The life course of schizophrenic
children. Biological Psychiatry 2: 165-172

Birmingham, D. (1962) Personal Communication

Black, J. and Scammell, (2005) *"Sleep and
Wakefullness"*,Stanford

Boorstin, D.J. (1983) *"The Discoverers"* Vintage
(1985), NY

Bornstein, B. (1951). On latency. Psychoanalytic Study
of the Child 6: 279-285. New York: International
Universities Press.

Boyesen, H. H. (1885) *"The Life of Goethe"* Kindle
(LOC-62)

Brook, Rupert, (1932) *"The Complete Poems of Rupert
Brook"* "THE CALL" (1905-1908) Available on Kindle

Butler, E.M. (1948) *"The Myth of the Magus"* Cambridge
University Press New York (page 121 ester.)

Cameron, Judy (2004) Interrelationships between
Hormones, Behavior, and Affect during Adolescence,
in Dahl, Ronald and Spear, Linda, Eds. (2004),
Annals of 4), Adolescent Brain Development, A
Period of Vulnerabilities and Opportunities,
in Dahl, Ronald and Spear, Linda, Eds. (2004),
"Annals of the New York Academy of Sciences" Vol
1021 p 1.

Campbell, J (1959) *"The Masks of God - PRIMITIVE
MYTHOLOGY"*, Viking Press, NY

Congreve, W. (1700) "The Way of the World" Dover, NY

Dahl, R. (2000) the New York Academy of Sciences Vol
   Dahl, R. (2004), Adolescent Brain Development,
   A Period of Vulnerabilities and Opportunities,
   in Dahl, Ronald and Spear, Linda, Eds. (2004),
   Annals of the New York Academy of Sciences Vol
   1021 p 1.

Damassio, A. R. (1999) "The Feeling of What Happens",
   New York, Harcourt Brace

Eggers, C. (1967). Prepubescent schizophrenia. Acta
   Paedopsychiatrica 34: 326-340.

Ferenczi, S. (1912) Dirigible Dreams, Zb. F. Psa 2,
   31, page 313-4

"During the process of waking up."

"We may add that these dreams are usually dreamt
   in the morning hours,..." [314]

Ferenczi, Sandor, (1913) Stages in he Development
   of the Sense of Reality, page 213 in 'Sex and
   Psychoanalysis", BasicFrankfortBooks (1950)

Flavell, J. H. (1963). The Developmental Psychology
   of Jean Piaget. New York: Van Nostrand, etal
   (1977)

Frankfort etal. (1977) "The Intellectual Adventure of
   Ancient Man" (p 386), Chicago University Press.,
   Chiicago

Freud, A. (1965) *"Normality and Pathology in Childhood"* IUP NY (1965) [See page 207]

Freud, S. (1897 Freud's Abstracts of his works # XXIV ON P 244 OF SE # III Hogarth, Press

Freud, S. (1905) *"The Interpretation of Dreams"* Hogarth Press

Freud, S.(1911) p 572 reference to the Marquis d'Hervey de Saint Denis, Quoted by Vaschide (1911) These people called Freud's attention to these dreams requiring the addition of a footnote. T. I.O. D.

Freud, S. (1909) Little Hans SE # 10 Hogarth Press London.

Freud, S. (1917) A Childhood Recollection from Dichtung und Wahrheit" SE # 17 Hogarth Press London.

Freud, S. (1926)*"Beyond the Pleasure Principle"*, S.E.18. pp. 419-439. London, Hogarth

Giedd, Jay (2004) Structural Magnetic Resonance Imaging of the Adolescent Brain, in Dahl, Ronald and Spear, Linda, Eds. (2004), Annals of the New York Academy of Sciences Vol 1021 P 77.

Goethe, J. (1774) *"The Sorrows of Young Werther"* Kindle loc. 7620 [24]

Goethe, J. (1782) "Ehrlenkoenig" Kindle loc. 11566 [33]

Goethe, J. (1790) *"Erotica Romana"* Kindle loc. 1039 [41]

Goethe, J. (1797) *"Hermann and Dorothea"* Kindle loc.10648 [48]

Goethe, J. (1808) *"Faust, Part 1"* Kindle loc. 0896 [59]

Goethe, J.(1810) *"Autobiography: Truth and Fiction Relating to My Life"* ("{DICTUM UND WAHRHEIT)"} kINDLE loc.12 [61]

Goethe, J. (1829) *"Wilhelm Meister, Years of Apprenticeship"* Vols. 2&3, Jon Calder, Pubs. Dallas 1978, Kindle. [80]

Goethe, J. (1833) *"Faust, Part 2"* Kindle loc --- [83]

Goldfarb, W. (1961). *"Childhood Schizophrenia"*, Boston: Harvard University Press

Grinn, H. (1880) *"The Life and Times of Goethe"* Kindle (Loc - 80)

Grunbaum, G.E. and Callois, Roger (1966) *The Dream In Human Societies"*, University of California Press. (1966)

Hampson, J. L., Hampson, J. G., and Money, J. (1959). "The syndrome of gonadal agenesis (ovarian agenesis) and male chromosomic patterns in girls and women." Bulletin of Johns Hopkins Hospital 97: 207 - 226.

Inhelder etal (1978) "Learning and the Development of Cognition",Journal of Psychological Anthropology, Vol.1, No. 2, page 255.

Jensen, A. K. (2015) "Johann Wolfgang von Goethe (1749-1832) in Internet Encyclopedia of Philosophy.

Jones, E. (1916) "The Theory of Symbolism" in "Papers on Psychoanalysis by Ernest Jones", Bailliere, Tindall and Cox, London (1950)

Jordan, K., and Prugh, D. (197]). Schizophreniform psychosis of late childhood. American Journal of Psychiatry 128: 323-329.

JOURNEY TO THE WEST, (1955) Foreign Languages Press, Beijing (1592)

Kelley, Ann etal (2004) Risk taking and Novelty Seeking in Adolescence, in in Dahl, Ronald and Spear, Linda, Eds. (2004), Annals of the New York Academy of Sciences

Klopstock, F. G (1748) "THE MESSIAH" KINDLE

Krystal, H. (1965) "Georgio De Chirico". AMERICAN IMAGO 22: 210-226

LaBerge, Stephan (1985) "Lucid Dreaming", Balantine. (1985)

Levy, E. z. (197]). Discussion of Jordan and Prugh. American Journal of Psychiatry 128: 329 - 392

Libbey, M.(1995) "The Primal Transference of the patient and the emotional position of the analyst: Thoughts on the analyst's work ego with the non-symbolizing patient", Presented to the 39th International Psychoanalytic Congress, Summarized on page 82 of the abstracts. San Francisco, 1995.

Luna, Betriz and Sweeney, John The Emergence of Collaborative Brain Function, in Dahl, Ronald and Spear, Linda, Eds. (2004), Annals of the New York Academy of Sciences Vol 1021 page 296.

Lopandin, V. M., and Stoyanov, S. (1970). Paraphrenia in adolescents with remittant schizophrenia. Korsakov Journal of Neuropsychiatry 70: 256-260.

Luria, A.R. (1972),*"The Man With A Shattered World"* Harvard (1987)

Mazzarello, G. P. (2010) Goethe, his love rivals and evidence of a generalized anxiety disorder in Humane Medicine Vol. 10, #3

Medina, John, and Pies, Ron (1999) The role of Seratonin in mediating the Effects of Atypical Antipsychotic Drugs, Psychiatric Times Monograph Supplement Sept 1999

Niobe The Myth (ANT) "Larousse Encyclopedia of Mythology", page 132, Prometheus Press, NY (1959)

O'Flaherty, Wendy Doniger (1982) The Dream Narrative and the Indian Doctrine of Illusion, Deadalus Vol 3. Number 3 Page 93

Philpot, Rex, and Kirstein, Cheryl (2004) Developmental Differences in the Accumbal Dopaminergic Response

to Repeated Ethanol Exposure, in Dahl, Ronald
and Spear, Linda, Eds. (2004), Annals of the New
York Academy of Sciences Vol 1021 P 422.

Piaget, J. (1945) *"Play Dreams and Imitation in
Childhood"*, NORTON (1946)

Piaget, J. (1960) *"THE CHILD'S CONCEPTION OF THE
WORLD"* Littlefield, Adams & Co. Paterson, NJ.

Plato (Ant) *"Phaedrus"* Hackett Publishers, Cambridge

Pompeiano, O. (1970) Mechanisms of Sensorimotor
integraton during Sleep. In Steller, E.& Sprague,
J.M. (Eds.), Progress in Physiolgical Psychology
Vol. 3, New York: Academic Press and

Robbins, T.W., Mehta, M.A, and Sahakian, B.J. (2000)
Boosting Working Memory. Science, Dec. 22, 2000.,
Page 2275

Rapaport, D., Ed. (1951) *"Organization and Pathology
Of Thought"* Columbia University Press, NY 1951

Rapoport, J. (1944). Fantasy Objects in children:
Psychoanalytic Review 31:316-321.

Roth, Thomas (2005) Characteristics and Determinants
of Normal Sleep, J. Clin Psychiatry 2004;65/Suppl
16/:8-11

Sakuntali, the mother of Bharata. in. *"Mahabarata"* And
Kalidasa's *"Sakuntali"* UNIVERSITY of CALIFORNIA
PRESS, BERKELEY, (1962)

Sarnoff, C.A. (1957) *"The Medical Aspects of Flying Motivation"*, SAMUSAF Publications, October 1957, 175 pages. Published by the United States Air Force for use as a textbook at the School of Aviation Medicine.

Sarnoff, C.A. and Mebane, J.C. (1958A) "Episodic G Force Intolerance", Journal of Aviation Medicine, April 1958, Vol. 29, pages 287-290.

Sarnoff, C.A. and Lamb, L.E. (1958B) "Significant Cardiac Arrhythmias Induced by Common Respiratory Maneuvers", American Journal of Cardiology, Vol. 2, No. 5, November 1958, pages 563-571.

Sarnoff, C.A. and Haberer, B.E. (1959) "The Technique of Studying Disturbances of Consciousness at Altitude", The Journal of Aviation Medicine, Vol. 30, April 1959, pages 231-240.

Sarnoff, C.A. and Silver, A., and Gottschalk, W., (1960) "Alcholism in Pregnancy", Psychiatric Quarterly, Vol. 34, July 1960, pages 461-471.

Sarnoff, C.A. (1963) Prepared Discussion (with Drs. Friend and Eidelberg) of paper "The Analysis of a Transvestite Boy" by Dr. Melitta Sperling, Abstract published in Psychoanalytic Quarterly, Vol. 32, No.2, 1963, page 471. [see reference to this in Freud, A. (1965)]

Sarnoff, C.A. (1965B) "A Contribution to the Understanding of the Concept 'The Universality of the Unconscious'", Abstracted in the Psychoanalytic Quarterly, Vol. 34, No. 2, 1965, pages 323-324.

Sarnoff, C.A. (1969A) "Slips of the Tongue in Child Analysis", Abstracted in Summaries of Scientific Papers, 56th Annual Meeting of the American Psychoanalytic Association, Vol. 2, May 1969, page 13.

Sarnoff, C.A. (1969B) "Mythic Symbols in Two Precolumbian Myths", American Imago, Vol. 26, No. 1, Spring, 1969.

Sarnoff, C.A. (1969C) "Psychiatric Problems, Childhood Emergencies", General Practice, Vol. 17, No. 45, Audio Digest Foundation, December 1, 1969.

Sarnoff, C.A. (1970A) "Mythic Symbols in Two Precolumbian Myths", American Imago, Vol. 26, 1969, Abstracted in Psychoanalytic Quarterly, Vol. 34, No. 2, April 1970, page 336.

Sarnoff, C.A. (1970B) "Symbols and Symptoms - A Case of Phytophobia in a Two Year Old Girl", the Psychoanalytic Quarterly, Vol. 39, No. 4, October 1970, pages 550-562.

Sarnoff, C.A. (1971). Ego structure in latency. The Psychoanalytic Quarterly 40: 387-412.

Sarnoff, C.A. June 8, 1971. Prepubescent sexuality. Medical Aspects of Human Sexuality 5: 122.

Sarnoff, C.A. _ (1972b). The vicissitudes of projection during the analysis of a girl in late latency-early adolescence. International Journal of Psycho-Analysis 53: 515.523.

Sarnoff, C.A. (1973a). Narcissism, adolescent masturbation fantasies and the search for reality. "Masturbation "From Infancy to Senescence", ed. Francis, J. J. etal, New York: International Universities Press, 1975.

Sarnoff, C.A. (1971A) "Transference in Children's Dreams", In Kanzer, M., The Unconscious Today, International Universities Press, New York, 1971, pages 436-441.

Sarnoff, C.A. (1971B) Discussion of Raskin, D. "Young Woman with Systemic Lupus with Psychiatric Complications", in Roche Report of Frontiers of Psychiatry, Vol. 1, No. 5, March 1, 1971.

Sarnoff, C.A. with Hart, M. (1971C) "The Impact of the Menarche", Journal of the American Academy of Child Psychiatry, Vol. 10, No. 2, April 1971, pages 257-271.

Sarnoff, C.A. (1971D) "Ego Structure in Latency", Psychoanalytic Quarterly, Vol. 40, No. 3, June 1971, pages 387-414.

Sarnoff, C.A. (1971F) "Prepubescent Sexuality", published in Medical Aspects of Human Sexuality, Vol. 5, No. 11, November 1971, page 124.

Sarnoff, C.A. (1972A) "Symbols in Shadows", a study of shadows in dreams, Journal of the American Psychoanalytic Association, Vol. 20, No. 1, January 1972, pages 59-91.

Sarnoff, C.A. (1972B) "The Ontogenesis of the System Consciousness - Part A. Fixation in the Abstract

System Consciousness", Abstracted in Summaries of Scientific Proceedings Annual Meeting of the American Psychoanalytic Association, Vol. 7, Annual 1972.

Sarnoff, C.A. (1972C) "The Meaning of William Rimmer's Flight and Pursuit'", The American Art Journal, Vol. 4, No. 2, page 18.

Sarnoff, C.A. (1972D) "The Vicissitudes of Projection During the Analysis of a Girl in Late Latency - Early Adolescence", The International Journal for Psychoanalysis, Part IV, 1972.

Sarnoff, C.A. (1972F), "A Psychiatric Evaluation of Increase in Sexual Drive of Somatic Origin", Accepted for publication in the Medical Aspect of Human Sexuality.

Sarnoff, C.A. (1973B) "Ontogenesis of the System Consciousness. Part B--Regressive Symbolization", Abstracted in the Summaries of Scientific Activities Annual Meeting of the American Psychoanalytic Association, Vol. 8, #Ann., p. 39.

Sarnoff, C.A. (1973C) "Narcissism, Adolescent Masturbation Fantasies and the Search for Reality", Abstracted in the Summaries of Scientific Activities Midwinter Meeting of the American Psychoanalytic Association.

Sarnoff, C.A. (1974) "Sonhos De Infancia. Aspectos Clinicos E Electroencefalograficos De Fenomenos Relacionados Ao Sono Na Infancia Precoce" in Temas Libres of the X Congresso Latino-Americano De

Psicanalise, pp. 521-541. "Dreams of Childhood", translated into Portuguese.

Sarnoff, C.A. (1975A) "Narcissism, Adolescent Masturbation Fantasies and the Search for Reality", in Marcus, I., and Francis, J. "Masturbation from Birth to Senescence, I.U.P., N.Y., 1975.

Sarnoff, C.A. (1976) *"Latency"*. Jason Aronson Inc. N.J., Publishers, May 1976.

Sarnoff, C.A. (1978) "Developmental Considerations in Psychotherapy of Latency Age Children", in the International Journal of Psychoanalytic Psychotherapy. Volume 7, Page 283, 1978

Sarnoff, C.A. (1978) "Lectures on Latency-1: Latency-An Expanding Psychiatric Horizon"

"Depression in Latency" Psychotherapy Tape Library 111 8th Avenue, New York, New York.

Sarnoff, C.A. (1979) "Latency" (Chapt. 5), in Bemporad, J.,"Child Development in Normality and Pathology". Bruner-Mazel. 1979.

Sarnoff, C.A. (1979) "The Influence of Myth on the Symbolic Forms Found in the Manifest Content of Dreams" (Abstract) in "Newsletter of the New Jersey Psychiatric Ass., Vol XIX, April 1979, No. 7, Page 3.

Sarnoff, C.A. (1980) Psychotherapy of the Latency Age Child," in Sholevar, G.P. et al., The Treatment of Emotional Disorders in Children and Adolescents. Spectrum Publishers, New York. In Print 1980.

Sarnoff, C.A. (1981) "Psychoanalysis and Personality Change" in "Academy Forum" Vol 25, Number 4 Winter 1981

Sarnoff, C.A. (1982) "Fathers in Latency" in Cath, Gurwitt, and Ross Eds "Father and Child" Little, Brown Inc Boston. 1982.

Sarnoff, C.A. (1982) "Derivatives of Latency"- Latency Origins of Symptoms of Anorexia Nervosa- in Wilson etal Eds. "The Fear of Being Fat" Aronson, N.Y. (1983).

Sarnoff, C.A. (1984) "Depression and Suicide in Children and Adolescents" in Guest Corner of the Postgraduate Center for Mental Health "NEWS" Vol 3 No. 2 Summer 1984. Pages 2 and 5.

Sarnoff, C.A.(1987) *"Psychotherapeutic Strategies During the Latency Years"* Jason Aronson Inc., N.J., Publishers Oct 1987

Sarnoff, C.A. (1987) *"Psychotherapeutic Strategies During Late Latency through Early Adolescence"* Jason Aronson Inc., N. J. Publishers Oct 1987

Sarnoff, C.A. (1988) "Memory, Symptoms, and Symbols" Chapter in Wilson, C.P. etal (eds) "Early Psychic Stress and Psychosomatic Disease", Aronson, N.J.

Sarnoff, C.A. (1988) "Adolescent Masochism" Chapter in Meyers and Glick (Eds) "Masochism: Current Psychoanalytic and Psychotherapeutic Contributions" The Analytic Press, Hillsdale, New Jersey.

Sarnoff, C.A. (1990) "Update on the Concept of the Neurotic Child", In Etezady (Ed) "The Neurotic Child", Aronson, Pubs.

Sarnoff, C.A. (1994) "Masochistic Braggadocio in "Adolescence" in American Psychoanalytic Association Publication - Cohen, T. & Etazady, M. H. (Eds)."The Vulnerable Child" International Universities Press.

Sarnoff, C.A. (1993) "The Role of Transference in Child Therapy" in M. Hossein Etazady (ed) "Treatment of the Neurotic Child" Jason Aronson, Publishers, N.J.

Sarnoff, C.A. (1993) "The Role of Play, Fantasy, and Dream in Child Therapy" in M. Hossein Etazady (Ed) "Treatment of the Neurotic Child" Jason Aronson Publishers, N.J.

Sarnoff, Charles (1995) "Current Practices and Procedures of Dynamic Psychotherapy with Children" CME article for DIRECTIONS IN PSYCHIATRY, The Hatherleigh Company Ltd.

Sarnoff, C. A. (1997) "Fantasies in the Grade School Years" in Kernberg, P. and Bemporad, J, (Eds) "The Grade School Child Section of "The Handbook of Child and Adolescent Psychiatry", John Wiley and Sons.

Sarnoff, C. A. (1997) "Cognitive Transformations in the Grade School Years" in Kernberg, P. and Bemporad, J, (Eds) "The Grade School Child

Section of "The Handbook of Child and Adolescent Psychiatry", John Wiley and Sons.

Sarnoff, C. A. (1997) "The Shift From Primary Process to Secondary Process Thinking" in Kernberg, P. and Bemporad, J, (Eds) "The Grade School Child Section of "The Handbook of Child and Adolescent Psychiatry", John Wiley and Sons.

Sarnoff, C. A. (1997) "The Shift From Preoperational Thinking to Concrete Operational Thinking" in Cherbourg, P. and Bemporad, J, (Eds) "The Grade School Child Section of "The Handbook of Child and Adolescent Psychiatry", John Wiley and Sons.

Sarnoff, C.A. (2002-2003) *"SYMBOLS IN STRUCTURE AND FUNCTION"*

VOLUME 1 "THEORIES OF SYMBOLISM" Philadelphia: *XLIBRIS 2002*

VOLUME 2 "SYMBOLS IN PSYCHOTHERAPY" Philadelphia: *XLIBRIS 2002*

VOLUME 3 "SYMBOLS IN CULTURE, ART, AND MYTH" Philadelphia: XLIBRIS 2003

Sarnoff, C. A. (2003) "Following Instincts" Bulletin of the Association for Psychoanalytic Medicine, Vol 38, Spring 2003. Page 40.

Sarnoff, C. A. (2007) *"The Feral Swan"*, (a novel) IUNIVERSE

Savary, L. M., Berne, P. H., and Williams, S. K.
(1984), "Dreams and Spiritual Growth" Paulist
Press, N.Y.

Schachtel, E. (1949) "On Memory and Childhood
Amnesia" in Schachtel, E. Ed. "Metamorphosis"
Basic Books NY 1959.

Siegel, Jerome (2004) The Nerurotransmitters of
Sleep, J clinical Psychiatry 2004;65 /suppl 16/:4-7.

Silberer, Herbert (1909) Report on a method of
Eliciting and Observing certain Symbolic
Hallucination Phenomena

Spengler, Oswald (1922) "Decline of the West", page
278 in volume2., Knopf (1928)

Sperling, M. (1952). Animal phobias in a two.year-old
child. Psychoanalytic Study of the Child 7: 115 -
125. New York: International Universities Press.

Sperling, M. (1974) "Dream Symbols and the
significance of their changes during analysis",
in "THE MAJOR NEUROSES AND BEHAVIOR DISORDERS IN
CHILDREN", JASON ARONSON. NY.

St. Augustine (400) "Confessions" IX, 24, Oxford,
London (1991)

St. Thomas Aquinas (1256-1259) "TRUTH" 3 volumes,
Chicago Regnery (1952-4)

Sterba, E. (J 949). Analysis of psychogenic
constipation in a two.year-old child. The

Psychoanalytic Studyof the Child 3/4: 227-252.
New York: International Universities Press.

Still, F. (900). Day terrors. Lancet 1: 292-294.

SUSSANA and the ELDERS (ANT) *"The Old Testament of
the Holy Bible"*. [Exodus3:12]

Stutte, H., and Dauner, I. (971). Systematized
delusions in early life schizophrenia. Journal
of Autism and Childhood Schizophrenia 1: 411-420.

Tamar, Widow of Onan (ANT) Genesis Chapter 38 *"Old
Testament"*

Thomas, L (1866) *"Mignon"* (an opera)

Von Grunbaum, G.E. and Callois, Roger (1966)
"The Dream In Human Societies", University of
California Press. (1966)

Walley Arthur (1919, 1942) "The Man Who Dreamed of
Fairies" by Po Chu-I in "Translatons from the
Chinese" Knopf page 1

Yahalom, I. (1967) 'Sense, Affect, and Image in
Development of the Symbolic Process' Int. J.
Psycho-Anal. (1967) 48, 373- 383.

Zweig, Stefan, (1926)" *"Beware of Pity"*, NEW YORK
REVIEW OF BOOKS

www.ingramcontent.com/pod-product-compliance
Lightning Source LLC
Chambersburg PA
CBHW020733180526
45163CB00001B/217